Fatty Liver Diet Cookbook

1000 Days of Healthy and Delicious Low-Fat Recipes to Heal Your Liver, Promote Energy and Live Healthy with 30 Days Meal Plan

Dr. Angela Wicks

Table of Contents

Introduction

Dietary fats are crucial for good health in general. These fats include linoleic acid, an essential fatty acid that supports a healthy metabolism and provides energy. Recent studies suggest that the consumption of unhealthy fats by an individual may be related to non-alcoholic fatty liver disease (NAFLD).

As the name suggests, fatty liver disease is a medical condition that is characterised by an abundance of fat in the liver. There are two kinds: those that are brought on by binge drinking and those that aren't. In the US, 5% of people have alcohol-related fatty liver disease.

Swelling in the abdomen, a rapid heartbeat, and extra weight around the waist are signs of fatty liver. The majority of diets for fatty liver include foods rich in polyunsaturated fats and vitamin B6. Elevated levels of cholesterol or triglycerides in the blood serum are one risk factor for non-alcoholic fatty liver disease that may be lessened by a low-carbohydrate diet.

Patients with non-alcoholic fatty liver disease are becoming more prevalent, but it is unclear what causes their condition.

The metabolic syndrome, a cluster of illnesses characterised by insulin resistance, dyslipidemia, and increases in body mass index, may be the main factor causing the accumulation of liver fat (BMI).

Due to the high fat content, eating diets high in unsaturated fatty acids has been linked to an elevated risk of non-alcoholic fatty liver disease (nearly 90%). Due to a lack of sufficient randomised trials, researchers are unable to determine whether the relationship between the two is causal or the result of confounding variables.

According to the American Liver Foundation, there is no medical treatment for non-alcoholic fatty liver disease. Making lifestyle changes, such as reducing weight, quitting alcohol, and eating foods low in saturated fat, is the best treatment for liver disease of any kind.

How Do You Get a Fatty Liver?

The liver is one of the most important organs in the body, responsible for filtering toxins, producing bile to help digest food, and regulating metabolism. One of the most common conditions that affects the liver is non-alcoholic fatty liver disease (NAFLD), which occurs when there is an excessive accumulation of fat in the liver cells. In this article, we will explore the causes and risk factors of fatty liver disease, the symptoms, diagnosis, treatment, and prevention of the condition.

Causes and Risk Factors of Fatty Liver Disease:
There are several causes and risk factors that can contribute to the development of fatty liver disease, including:

Obesity: One of the main risk factors for NAFLD is obesity, which can cause an accumulation of fat in the liver cells. People who are overweight or obese are more likely to develop NAFLD than those who maintain a healthy weight.

Insulin resistance: Insulin resistance is another risk factor for NAFLD, as it can lead to an accumulation of fat in the liver cells. Insulin resistance is a condition where the body is unable to use insulin properly, which can lead to high blood sugar levels.

Type 2 diabetes: People with type 2 diabetes are more likely to develop NAFLD, as the condition is closely linked to insulin resistance and high blood sugar levels.

High cholesterol and triglycerides: High levels of cholesterol and triglycerides in the blood can also contribute to the development of NAFLD, as they can lead to an accumulation of fat in the liver cells.

Metabolic syndrome: Metabolic syndrome is a group of conditions that are often associated with obesity, including high blood pressure, high blood sugar, high cholesterol levels, and excess belly fat. People with metabolic syndrome are at a higher risk of developing NAFLD.

Rapid weight loss: Rapid weight loss can also contribute to the development of NAFLD, as the body may break down fat stores in the liver, leading to an accumulation of fat in the liver cells.

Medications: Certain medications, such as corticosteroids, tamoxifen, and methotrexate, can also contribute to the development of NAFLD.

Considerable Risk Factors

Additionally, fatty liver is linked to several other risk factors, including:
- Insulin resistance
- A greater accumulation of visceral fat
- Autoimmune illnesses
- Deficiency in nutrients (especially insufficient intake of protein)
- Diabetic liver disease
- Excessive sugar intake
- Genetic factors
- Insufficiency of insulin
- Lifestyles that are too passive
- Obesity
- Old age
- Several narcotics and environmental contaminants

Symptoms of Fatty Liver

The usual for people with fatty liver disease is either no symptoms or very specific digestive problems. The following signs and symptoms frequently indicate fatty liver:

• Difficulty concentrating;
• Bloating
• A decrease in production
• Feeling of right upper abdominal pressure

Early signs of the condition don't include symptoms like nausea, vomiting, or pain in the right upper abdomen around the liver. The eyes and skin may become yellow if liver function is already gravely impaired.

We suggest that you see your primary healthcare provider or a doctor if you have any of these symptoms. They will first talk about your symptoms and do a physical examination. While palpable, diseases other than fatty liver may be to blame for liver growth. As a result, a blood test to check the liver's levels is typically done afterwards. The liver might operate improperly despite its normal levels, or vice versa. As a consequence, when the surgery is over, your family doctor will schedule an ultrasound with you. This scan will clearly reveal the accumulation of fat in the liver, showing how far along it is. The liver is regarded as fatty when its fat content exceeds 5% of its total weight (the weight of a healthy liver is between 1500 and 2000 grammes in an adult). In some cases, your doctor might tell you to find a specialist who can take a small sample of your liver cells to get a better idea of how healthy they are.

Types of Fatty Liver Disease

Liver Failure

Liver failure is a serious medical condition that occurs when the liver is unable to perform its normal functions. The liver is responsible for filtering toxins from the blood, producing bile to aid in digestion, storing vitamins and minerals, and regulating blood clotting. When the liver fails, these functions are impaired, which can lead to a wide range of symptoms and complications.

Liver failure can be acute or chronic. Acute liver failure occurs rapidly, often within a few days or weeks, and can be caused by infections, drug overdose, or acute viral hepatitis. Chronic liver failure develops over a longer period of time, usually years, and is often caused by chronic viral hepatitis, alcohol abuse, or non-alcoholic fatty liver disease.

Symptoms of liver failure can include jaundice (yellowing of the skin and eyes), abdominal swelling and pain, fatigue, confusion, and easy bruising or bleeding. In severe cases, liver failure can lead to coma and death.

Treatment for liver failure depends on the underlying cause and the severity of the condition. In some cases, supportive care such as fluids, electrolytes, and nutrition may be enough to allow the liver to recover. In other cases, liver transplantation may be necessary.

Prevention of liver failure involves avoiding excessive alcohol consumption, practicing safe sex, getting vaccinated against hepatitis B and C, and avoiding exposure to toxic substances. If you have any symptoms of liver failure, it's important to see a doctor right away.

Liver Cancer

Liver cancer, also known as hepatocellular carcinoma (HCC), is a type of cancer that starts in the liver. It is the sixth most common cancer in the world and the fourth leading cause of cancer-related deaths.

The liver is a vital organ in the body that performs several essential functions, including filtering toxins and waste products from the blood, producing bile to aid in digestion, and regulating metabolism. When liver cells begin to grow abnormally and uncontrollably, they can form a tumor that can invade nearby tissues and spread to other parts of the body.

The risk factors for liver cancer include chronic infection with hepatitis B or C, cirrhosis of the liver, excessive alcohol consumption, obesity, diabetes, and exposure to certain chemicals and toxins. Symptoms of liver cancer may include abdominal pain and swelling, fatigue, unexplained weight loss, loss of appetite, and yellowing of the skin and eyes (jaundice).

Treatment options for liver cancer depend on the stage and severity of the cancer, as well as the patient's overall health. Treatment may include surgery to remove the tumor, liver transplant, chemotherapy, radiation therapy, or a combination of these approaches. In some cases, targeted therapies and immunotherapy may also be used to treat liver cancer.

It is important to note that early detection and treatment of liver cancer can improve the chances of a successful outcome. Regular screening and monitoring for liver cancer are recommended for individuals who are at high risk, such as those with chronic liver disease or a history of hepatitis B or C infection.

Alcoholic Liver Disease (ALD

Alcoholic liver disease (ALD) is a term used to describe the damage caused to the liver as a result of prolonged and excessive alcohol consumption. The liver is the largest organ in the human body and is responsible for numerous vital functions, including filtering toxins from the blood, producing bile, and storing energy in the form of glycogen. When alcohol is consumed in excess, it can have a significant impact on the liver's ability to function correctly, leading to a range of serious health problems.

The development of ALD is linked to the amount and frequency of alcohol consumption. Prolonged and excessive drinking can lead to the accumulation of fat in the liver, a condition known as fatty liver. This condition is reversible with abstinence from alcohol, but if alcohol consumption continues, it can progress to a more severe form of liver damage known as alcoholic hepatitis. In the later stages of ALD, the liver can become permanently scarred, leading to a condition known as cirrhosis.

Symptoms of ALD vary depending on the stage of the disease. In the early stages, there may be no noticeable symptoms, but as the disease progresses, symptoms can include:
- Fatigue
- Nausea
- Loss of appetite
- Abdominal pain and swelling
- Jaundice (yellowing of the skin and eyes)
- Swelling in the legs and ankles
- Confusion and difficulty thinking clearly

In severe cases of alcoholic hepatitis and cirrhosis, the liver may stop functioning altogether, leading to life-threatening complications such as internal bleeding, kidney failure, and liver cancer.

The diagnosis of ALD is typically made through a combination of physical examination, blood tests, and imaging studies such as ultrasound, CT scan, or MRI. A liver biopsy may also be performed to assess the extent of liver damage.

The treatment of ALD depends on the stage of the disease. In the early stages, the primary treatment is abstinence from alcohol. This can help to reverse the damage caused to the liver and prevent the disease from progressing. In more advanced stages of the disease, other treatments may be necessary, such as medication to reduce inflammation and swelling in the liver, and in some cases, liver transplantation.

Preventing ALD involves avoiding or limiting alcohol consumption. The recommended limits for alcohol consumption are no more than 14 units per week for men and women, spread out over several days. Binge drinking, defined as consuming more than six units in one sitting, should be avoided entirely.

The long-term consequences of ALD can be severe, with a significant impact on the quality of life and life expectancy of those affected. Complications such as liver failure and liver cancer can be life-threatening, and there is no cure for advanced stages of the disease.

In conclusion, ALD is a serious and potentially life-threatening condition that is caused by prolonged and excessive alcohol consumption. The disease progresses through stages, with early diagnosis and treatment being essential to prevent further damage to the liver. Prevention through limiting or avoiding alcohol consumption is key to reducing the risk of developing ALD. For those already affected by the disease, abstinence from alcohol is crucial to prevent further damage and potentially reverse some of the existing damage to the liver.

Acute Viral Hepatitis

Acute viral hepatitis is a medical condition that is caused by viral infections that attack the liver. It is a significant public health issue that affects millions of people globally, with a high mortality rate if left untreated. In this article, we will discuss the different types of acute viral hepatitis, their causes, symptoms, diagnosis, treatment, and prevention.

Types of Acute Viral Hepatitis:
There are five main types of viral hepatitis: A, B, C, D, and E. Each type is caused by a different virus and has different symptoms and treatment methods.

Hepatitis A:
Hepatitis A is a highly contagious virus that spreads through contaminated food or water, or close personal contact with an infected person. The virus usually resolves on its own within a few weeks, and most people recover fully with no long-term effects. Symptoms of hepatitis A include fever, fatigue, loss of appetite, nausea, vomiting, abdominal pain, dark urine, and yellowing of the skin and eyes.

Hepatitis B:
Hepatitis B is a viral infection that spreads through contact with infected blood, semen, or other body fluids. The virus can also spread from mother to child during childbirth. Symptoms of hepatitis B include fatigue, nausea, vomiting, abdominal pain, joint pain, and jaundice. In some cases, hepatitis B can become chronic, leading to liver damage, liver failure, and liver cancer.

Hepatitis C:
Hepatitis C is a viral infection that spreads through contact with infected blood. It is a leading cause of liver disease and liver cancer. Symptoms of hepatitis C include fatigue, nausea, vomiting,

abdominal pain, joint pain, and jaundice. Most people with hepatitis C develop chronic hepatitis, which can lead to liver cirrhosis, liver failure, and liver cancer.

Hepatitis D:
Hepatitis D is a viral infection that occurs only in people who are already infected with hepatitis B. The virus can only replicate in the presence of the hepatitis B virus. Symptoms of hepatitis D are similar to those of hepatitis B.

Hepatitis E:
Hepatitis E is a viral infection that spreads through contaminated food or water, especially in areas with poor sanitation. Symptoms of hepatitis E include fever, fatigue, loss of appetite, nausea, vomiting, abdominal pain, dark urine, and yellowing of the skin and eyes.

Causes of Acute Viral Hepatitis:
Acute viral hepatitis is caused by a group of viruses that attack the liver. The most common causes of acute viral hepatitis are hepatitis A, B, and C. These viruses spread through contaminated food or water, contact with infected blood or other body fluids, or close personal contact with an infected person.

Risk Factors:
Certain factors increase the risk of developing acute viral hepatitis. These include:

- Having unprotected sex with an infected person.
- Sharing needles, syringes, or other drug equipment with an infected person.
- Living in or traveling to areas with poor sanitation and hygiene.
- Eating contaminated food or drinking contaminated water.

- Having a weakened immune system due to HIV, cancer, or other conditions.

Symptoms of Acute Viral Hepatitis:
The symptoms of acute viral hepatitis can vary depending on the type of virus and the severity of the infection. However, some common symptoms include:

- Fatigue
- Nausea
- Vomiting
- Abdominal pain
- Loss of appetite
- Joint pain
- Jaundice (yellowing of the skin and eyes)
- Dark urine
- Clay-colored stools

Diagnosis of Acute Viral Hepatitis:
To diagnose acute viral hepatitis, your doctor will perform a physical exam and ask about your symptoms and medical history. They may also order blood tests to check for the presence of the virus and assess liver function.

Non-Alcoholic Fatty Liver Disease (NAFLD)

Non-alcoholic fatty liver disease (NAFLD) is a condition that is characterized by an accumulation of fat in the liver cells, also known as hepatocytes, in people who drink little to no alcohol. It is the most common liver disease in the Western world and affects an estimated 25% of the global population. NAFLD is strongly associated with obesity, insulin resistance, and metabolic syndrome, which are all conditions that increase the risk of cardiovascular disease and type 2 diabetes.

NAFLD can be divided into two types: simple fatty liver (also known as non-alcoholic fatty liver, or NAFL) and non-alcoholic steatohepatitis (NASH). NAFL is the less severe form and is characterized by the accumulation of fat in the liver cells without any inflammation or damage. NASH, on the other hand, is a more serious condition that is characterized by the accumulation of fat in the liver cells along with inflammation and damage. NASH can lead to cirrhosis and liver failure, and it is the second leading cause of liver transplantation in the United States.

The exact cause of NAFLD is not known, but it is believed to be related to insulin resistance, which occurs when the body's cells do not respond normally to insulin. Insulin is a hormone that regulates blood sugar levels, and when cells become resistant to its effects, the body produces more insulin to compensate. This can lead to an increase in the production of fat by the liver, as well as an increase in the accumulation of fat in the liver cells.

NAFLD is also associated with other risk factors, such as obesity, type 2 diabetes, high blood pressure, high cholesterol, and metabolic syndrome. These conditions are all related to insulin resistance and are common in people with NAFLD. In addition, certain medications, such as corticosteroids and tamoxifen, as well as some viral infections, such as hepatitis C, can increase the risk of NAFLD.

The symptoms of NAFLD are usually mild or absent, especially in the early stages. However, as the disease progresses, symptoms may include fatigue, abdominal discomfort, and enlarged liver. NASH, in particular, can cause more severe symptoms, such as jaundice, itching, and easy bruising or bleeding.

The diagnosis of NAFLD is typically made through blood tests, imaging tests, and liver biopsy. Blood tests can detect elevated liver enzymes, which can indicate liver damage, as well as high levels of insulin and glucose, which can indicate insulin resistance. Imaging tests, such as ultrasound, CT scan, or MRI, can show the accumulation of fat in the liver. A liver biopsy involves removing a small sample of liver tissue for examination under a microscope to look for signs of inflammation and damage.

The treatment of NAFLD involves lifestyle changes and, in some cases, medication. The most important lifestyle changes include weight loss, exercise, and a healthy diet. Even a modest weight loss of 5-10% can improve liver function and reduce the accumulation of fat in the liver cells. Exercise, particularly aerobic exercise, can also improve insulin sensitivity and reduce liver fat. A healthy diet should include plenty of fruits, vegetables, whole grains, and lean protein, and should limit saturated and trans fats, added sugars, and refined carbohydrates.

There are also several medications that may be used to treat NAFLD, although none are currently approved specifically for this condition. These include drugs that improve insulin sensitivity, such as metformin and thiazolidinediones, and drugs that reduce liver fat, such as vitamin E and pioglitazone. However, these medications have not been extensively studied for the treatment of NAFLD, and their long-term safety and effectiveness are not well understood.

Chronic Viral Hepatitis

Chronic Viral Hepatitis is a condition where the liver becomes inflamed and damaged due to a viral infection that persists for more than six months. There are five types of viral hepatitis, but the most common types that can lead to chronic infection are hepatitis B virus (HBV) and hepatitis C virus (HCV).

Hepatitis B virus is transmitted through blood, semen, or other bodily fluids and is endemic in many parts of the world, especially in Africa, Asia, and the Pacific Islands. In contrast, hepatitis C virus is primarily transmitted through blood, and the most common mode of transmission is through the use of contaminated needles or syringes, as well as through blood transfusions or organ transplants before the introduction of screening tests.

Symptoms of chronic viral hepatitis may not be noticeable for many years, as the disease progresses slowly and gradually. Symptoms may include fatigue, weakness, loss of appetite, abdominal pain, jaundice, and liver cirrhosis or cancer.
Chronic viral hepatitis is diagnosed through blood tests that measure the levels of liver enzymes and antibodies against the virus. In some cases, a liver biopsy may be required to confirm the diagnosis and assess the degree of liver damage.

Treatment of chronic viral hepatitis depends on the type of virus and the degree of liver damage. Antiviral medications are available for both HBV and HCV, and they are used to reduce viral replication, prevent the progression of liver damage, and improve overall liver function. However, these medications are not always effective, and some patients may require long-term treatment or even liver transplantation.

Prevention of chronic viral hepatitis involves the use of safe sex practices, avoiding sharing needles or other equipment that may come in contact with blood, and vaccination against hepatitis B. There is currently no vaccine for hepatitis C, but early diagnosis and treatment can help prevent chronic infection.

Chronic viral hepatitis can have significant long-term consequences if left untreated. It can lead to liver cirrhosis, liver failure, and even liver cancer. Therefore, early detection and treatment are critical to preventing these complications.

In conclusion, chronic viral hepatitis is a serious and potentially life-threatening condition that can result from an infection with either hepatitis B or C virus. It is a slow and gradual disease that may not present noticeable symptoms for many years, and early detection and treatment are essential to prevent long-term complications. Preventive measures such as vaccination and safe sex practices can also help reduce the risk of infection.

Autoimmune Hepatitis

Autoimmune hepatitis (AIH) is a rare autoimmune liver disease that occurs when the body's immune system mistakenly attacks healthy liver cells, leading to inflammation and damage. The disease is characterized by elevated liver enzymes, which can lead to liver damage, cirrhosis, and even liver failure if left untreated. In this article, we will discuss the causes, symptoms, diagnosis, and treatment of autoimmune hepatitis in detail.

Causes:
The exact cause of AIH is not known, but research suggests that a combination of genetic and environmental factors may trigger an immune response that attacks the liver. Some risk factors that may contribute to the development of AIH include:

- **Genetics:** People with a family history of autoimmune diseases are more likely to develop AIH.
- **Environmental factors:** Exposure to toxins, viruses, or medications may trigger an autoimmune response in susceptible individuals.

- **Gender:** Women are more likely to develop AIH than men.
- Age: AIH can occur at any age, but it most commonly affects people between the ages of 15 and 40.

Symptoms:

The symptoms of AIH can vary widely, and some people may have no symptoms at all. The most common symptoms of AIH include:

- **Fatigue:** Chronic fatigue is one of the most common symptoms of AIH.
- **Abdominal pain:** Pain in the upper right quadrant of the abdomen is common.
- **Jaundice:** Yellowing of the skin and eyes due to elevated bilirubin levels.
- **Nausea and vomiting:** These symptoms may occur due to liver dysfunction.
- **Loss of appetite:** A decrease in appetite may occur due to nausea and abdominal pain.
- **Joint pain:** Some people with AIH may experience joint pain and swelling.
- **Enlarged liver and spleen:** The liver and spleen may become enlarged due to inflammation.

Diagnosis:

The diagnosis of AIH is based on a combination of clinical, laboratory, and histological criteria. The diagnostic process may include the following tests:

- **Blood tests:** Elevated liver enzymes, such as ALT and AST, are the most common findings in people with AIH.
- **Serology**: The presence of specific antibodies, such as anti-nuclear antibody (ANA) and anti-smooth muscle antibody (ASMA), may be used to support the diagnosis.

- **Liver biopsy:** A liver biopsy may be performed to confirm the diagnosis and assess the degree of liver damage.
- **Imaging tests:** Ultrasound, CT scan, or MRI may be used to assess the liver and other organs.

Treatment:

The goal of treatment for AIH is to suppress the immune system and reduce inflammation in the liver. The standard treatment for AIH involves the use of corticosteroids, such as prednisone, and immunosuppressive drugs, such as azathioprine. The treatment may also include:

- **Monitoring liver function:** Regular blood tests may be used to monitor liver function and adjust the dosage of medications as needed.
- **Nutrition support:** A healthy diet, including adequate protein and calorie intake, is important for people with AIH.
- **Avoidance of triggers:** Certain medications, such as acetaminophen and nonsteroidal anti-inflammatory drugs (NSAIDs), should be avoided as they can worsen liver damage.
- **Liver transplant:** In severe cases of AIH, liver transplant may be necessary to prevent liver failure.

Prognosis:

The prognosis for AIH varies depending on the severity of the disease and the response to treatment. With appropriate treatment, most people with AIH can achieve remission and have a normal life expectancy. However, some people may experience relapses or develop complications, such as cirrhosis or liver failure, despite treatment.

Detox Your Body

While physicians often state, "You can't detox your strong liver as it already detoxifies itself," liver detox is contentious.

This may be the case; however, keep in mind that toxins intended for breakdown are among the toxins that are overproduced by a fatty liver. Nevertheless, the liver cannot carry out its duty because of the fat deposits.

Each person's body goes through detoxification procedures that are crucial to their health and wellness. These steps are necessary to get rid of dangerous chemicals that could stop different organ systems from working as they should.Most people need detox because they are exposed to bad cleaning products, pollution, and processed foods.

In the event of a fatty liver, liver detoxification is also advantageous. In this instance, the liver has to be restarted since it has lost all of its functional abilities. The liver may effectively start again via detoxification. The process boosts the performance and functionalities of the device, similar to tuning and cleaning the spark plug of an automobile. Adopting a nutritious diet also helps your body's detoxification processes and reduces its exposure to potentially dangerous toxins.

The process of liver cleaning, or detoxification, is not simple. You can feel weak and have frequent hunger pangs. It's not an impossible job, however. There are many purging diets that may aid with fatty liver, but they all seem to follow the same pattern. You must abstain from all harmful foods when following a liver-cleansing diet. It entails drinking juice or a certain tea for a predetermined amount of time—up to 10 days.

If you eat less every day and don't eat unhealthy meals, it might help the liver get rid of all the poisonous and harmful chemicals in your body.This is particularly helpful in the context of fatty liver, where defects in liver function have led to the accumulation of toxic chemicals, aggravating the illness.

You'll often hear folks caution you about the harmful consequences of liver-cleansing diets. Potential side effects include low blood sugar, poor energy, weariness, muscular pain, dizziness, and nausea. Although following such a diet may alter certain aspects of your regular routine, the idea that a liver cleanse is bad for your general health is essentially false. This allows the diet to be customized to meet the specific needs and requirements of each individual.

If you want to stick to a liver detox diet, you need to know what other foods you can eat. From breakfast to daily snacks, everything is laid out in a way that makes it easy to lose weight quickly and treat fatty liver without putting your health at risk.

This section has an easy-to-find list of the foods that should still make up most of your diet.

Foods to Enjoy

- Legumes: The greatest foods for regulating blood sugar and fat levels include lentils, chickpeas, black beans, navy beans, pinto beans, kidney beans, and their cousins. Due to the relatively high levels of protein and fiber in these meals, they are also very satisfying.
- Fruit: Fruits of all sorts are effective because they are high in fiber, vitamins, minerals, anti-inflammatory polyphenol chemicals, and other nutrients. There is no need to choose a side when it comes to fruit; however, berries, oranges, apples, and bananas may be particularly healthy.
- Vegetables are very good for your health because they have a lot of fiber, vitamins, minerals, and antioxidants. Vegetables must play a significant role in your nutritional plan.

- Non-starchy vegetables: these include Brussels sprouts, broccoli, cauliflower, bell peppers, spinach, kale, asparagus, Swiss chard, and zucchini.
- starchy vegetables, such as sweet potatoes, squash of all varieties, and beets
- Lean Meats (Chicken, Turkey, Especially Breast): Lean meats, such as chicken and turkey breast, are a great way to receive protein without the saturated fat found in other meats.
- Foods high in healthy fats (such as nuts, seeds, avocado, and certain oils): These foods are always a good choice. High-omega-3-fat foods include walnuts, chia, hemp, and flax seeds. Saturated fats have the opposite impact as avocado and olive oil. The monounsaturated fat content is high. Other foods rich in this fat include cashews, almonds, and pistachios. They also contain significant amounts of fat-soluble vitamin E, which may be particularly advantageous for liver health and cholesterol reduction.
- Eggs: Contrary to popular belief, they may be consumed often. As long as you consume them as part of a balanced diet, their cholesterol level won't hurt you.
- Grains with a low or medium glycemic index: People with fatty liver should choose grains with a low glycemic index (GI). This is because insulin resistance and type 2 diabetes may make the condition worse. This group of foods includes brown rice, whole grain bread or pasta, quinoa, steel-cut oats, and quinoa.
- Soy: Foods made from soy, such as tofu, tempeh, soy milk, and edamame, provide an alternative protein source that may help you rely less on animal proteins that are high in saturated fats, which will benefit the health of your liver. Foods containing soy have a definite reducing impact on cholesterol.
- Low-fat dairy products, such as yogurt and kefir, which are high in probiotics.

- Fatty Fish and Seafood Varieties: Salmon, mackerel, trout, tuna, and sardines are some fish that are rich in omega-3 fatty acids and vitamin D.

Breakfast

Poblano Fritatta

Preparation time: 10 minutes
Cooking time: 15 minutes
Servings: 4
Ingredients:
- 5 eggs, beaten
- 1 poblano chile, chopped, raw
- 1 oz scallions, chopped
- 1/3 cup heavy cream
- ½ teaspoon butter
- ½ teaspoon salt
- ½ teaspoon chili flakes
- 1 tablespoon fresh cilantro, chopped

Directions:
1. Whisk eggs and heavy cream together until well combined. Add salt, chili flakes, scallions, sliced poblano chiles, and fresh cilantro. Melt the butter by placing it in the skillet.
2. Add egg mixture and, if necessary, flatten it in the skillet. Over a medium-low heat, cover the pan and cook the frittata for 15 minutes. The frittata will be firm once it has finished cooking.
Nutrition:
Calories: 131, Fat: 10.4, Carbs: 1.3, Protein: 8.2

Corn and Shrimp Salad

Preparation time: 10 minutes
Cooking time: 10 minutes
Servings: 4
Ingredients:
- 4 ears of sweet corn, husked
- 1 avocado, peeled, pitted and chopped

- ½ cup basil, chopped
- A pinch of salt and black pepper
- 1 pound shrimp, peeled and deveined
- 1 and ½ cups cherry tomatoes, halved
- ¼ cup olive oil

Directions:

1. Place the corn in a pot, cover with water, and cook over medium heat for 6 minutes. Drain, let cool, then chop the corn from the cob and place it in a bowl.

2. Skewer the shrimp and brush them with some of the oil. Put the skewers on the prepared grill and cook for 2 minutes on each side over medium heat. Then take from the skewers and place over the corn.

3. Toss in the remaining ingredients, then divide the mixture among plates and serve as breakfast.

Nutrition:

Calories: 371, Fat: 22, Carbs: 25, Protein: 23

Tuna Salad

Preparation time: 10 minutes

Cooking time: 0 minutes

Servings: 2

Ingredients:

- 12 ounces canned tuna in water, drained and flaked
- ¼ cup roasted red peppers, chopped
- 2 tablespoons capers, drained
- 8 kalamata olives, pitted and sliced
- 2 tablespoons olive oil tablespoon parsley, chopped
- 1 tablespoon lemon juice
- A pinch of salt and black pepper

Directions:

1. Toss the tuna with the remaining ingredients in a bowl, then divide the mixture among plates and serve as breakfast.

Nutrition:
Calories: 250, Fat: 17.3, Carbs: 2.7, Protein: 10.1

Mushroom-Egg Casserole

Preparation time: 7 minutes
Cooking time: 25 minutes
Servings: 3
Ingredients:

- ½ cup mushrooms, chopped
- ½ yellow onion, diced
- 4 eggs, beaten
- 1 tablespoon coconut flakes
- ½ teaspoon chili pepper
- 1 oz Cheddar cheese, shredded
- 1 teaspoon canola oil

Directions:
1. Fill the skillet with canola oil and heat it well. Add the mushrooms and onion, and roast the vegetables for 5-8 minutes, or until they are tender-crisp.
2. Place the prepared vegetables in the casserole dish. Add Cheddar cheese, chile pepper, and coconut flakes.
3. Then, thoroughly stir in the eggs. At 360°F, bake the casserole for 15 minutes.
Nutrition:
Calories: 152, Fat: 11.1, Carbs: 3, Protein: 10.4

Tomato and Lentils Salad

Preparation time: 10 minutes
Cooking time: 35 minutes
Servings: 4
Ingredients:

- 2 yellow onions, chopped
- 4 garlic cloves, minced

- 2 cups brown lentils
- 1 tablespoon olive oil
- A pinch of salt and black pepper
- ½ teaspoon sweet paprika
- ½ teaspoon ginger, grated
- 3 cups water
- ¼ cup lemon juice
- ¾ cup Greek yogurt
- 3 tablespoons tomato paste

Directions:
1. In a pot with the oil already heated to medium-high, add the onions and cook for 2 minutes. Stir in the lentils and garlic, then continue cooking for an additional minute. Cook for 30 minutes with the lid on after adding the water and bringing to a simmer.
2. Combine the remaining ingredients—aside from the yogurt—with the lemon juice. Toss, portion the mixture into bowls, add the yogurt on top, and then serve.

Nutrition:
Calories: 294, Fat: 3, Carbs: 49, Protein: 21

Walnuts Yogurt Mix

Preparation time: 10 minutes
Cooking time: 0 minutes
Servings: 6

Ingredients:
- 2 ½ cups Greek yogurt
- 1 ½ cups walnuts, chopped
- 1 teaspoon vanilla extract
- ¾ cup honey
- 2 teaspoons cinnamon powder

Directions:

1. Toss the yoghurt with the walnuts and the other ingredients in a dish, then divide the mixture into smaller portions and refrigerate for 10 minutes before serving as breakfast.

Nutrition:

Calories: 388, Fat: 24.6, Carbs: 39.1, Protein: 10.2

Vegetable Breakfast Bowl

Preparation time: 10 minutes

Cooking time: 35 minutes

Servings: 4

Ingredients:

- 1 cup sweet potatoes, peeled, chopped
- 1 russet potato, chopped
- 1 red onion, sliced
- 2 bell pepper, trimmed
- ½ teaspoon garlic powder
- ¾ teaspoon onion powder
- 1 tablespoon olive oil
- 1 tablespoon Sriracha sauce
- 1 tablespoon coconut milk

Directions:

1. Use baking paper to line the baking pan. Put the sweet potato and russet potatoes, both chopped, in the tray. Add the onion, bell peppers, and season the veggies with the onion, garlic, and olive oil. With the aid of your fingers, thoroughly combine the veggies, then place them in the oven that has been preheated to 360°F.

2. For 45 minutes, bake the veggies. Make the sauce in the meanwhile by combining Sriracha sauce and coconut milk. Add Sriracha sauce to the cooked veggies before placing them on serving dishes.

Nutrition:

Calories: 213, Fat: 7.2, Carbs: 34.6, Protein: 3.6

Couscous and Chickpeas Bowls

Preparation time: 10 minutes
Cooking time: 6 minutes
Servings: 4

Ingredients:

- ¾ cup whole wheat couscous
- 1 yellow onion, chopped
- 1 tablespoon olive oil
- 1 cup water
- 2 garlic cloves, minced
- 15 ounces canned chickpeas, drained and rinsed
- A pinch of salt and black pepper
- 15 ounces canned tomatoes, chopped
- 14 ounces canned artichokes, drained and chopped
- ½ cup Greek olives, pitted and chopped
- ½ teaspoon oregano, dried
- 1 tablespoon lemon juice

Directions:

1. In a medium-sized saucepan, add the water, bring to a boil, whisk in the couscous, remove from the heat, cover the pan, and let stand for 10 minutes before fluffing with a fork.
2. Add the onion to a pan that has oil in it and cook for 2 minutes over medium-high heat.
3. Add the other ingredients, stir, and cook for an additional 4 minutes. For breakfast, mix in the couscous, divide it into bowls, and serve.

Nutrition:

Calories: 340, Fat: 10, Carbs: 51, Protein: 11

Lemon Peas Quinoa Mix

Preparation time: 10 minutes
Cooking time: 20 minutes

Servings: 4
Ingredients:

- 1 ½ cups quinoa, rinsed pound asparagus, steamed and chopped
- 3 cups water tablespoons parsley, chopped
- 2 tablespoons lemon juice
- 1 teaspoon lemon zest, grated
- ½ pound snap peas, steamed
- ½ pound green beans, trimmed and halved
- A pinch of salt and black pepper
- 3 tablespoons pumpkin seeds
- 1 cup cherry tomatoes, halved
- 2 tablespoons olive oil

Directions:

1. Add the quinoa to the boiling water in a saucepan, stir, and cook for 20 minutes over medium heat.
2. Toss the quinoa with the other ingredients, including the parsley and lemon juice, then divide the mixture among plates and serve as breakfast.

Nutrition:

Calories: 417, Fat: 15, Carbs: 58, Protein: 16

Breakfast Green Smoothie

Preparation time: 7 minutes
Cooking time: 0 minutes
Servings: 2
Ingredients:

- 2 cups spinach
- 2 cups kale
- 1 cup bok choy
- 1 ½ cup organic almond milk
- 1 tablespoon almonds, chopped

- ½ cup of water

Directions:

1. Add all ingredients to a blender and process until a smooth slurry is obtained. Place the serving cups with the smoothie inside.
2. If desired, add ice cubes.

Nutrition:

Calories: 107, Fat: 3.6, Carbs: 15.5, Protein: 4.8

Brown Rice Salad

Preparation time: 10 minutes
Cooking time: 0 minutes
Servings: 4

Ingredients:

- 9 ounces brown rice, cooked
- 7 cups baby arugula
- 15 ounces canned garbanzo beans, drained and rinsed
- 4 ounces feta cheese, crumbled
- ¾ cup basil, chopped
- A pinch of salt and black pepper
- 2 tablespoons lemon juice
- ¼ teaspoon lemon zest, grated
- ¼ cup olive oil

Directions:

1. Toss the brown rice, arugula, beans, and the other ingredients in a salad dish before serving cold as breakfast.

Nutrition:

Calories: 473, Fat: 22, Carbs: 53, Protein: 13

Tahini Pine Nuts Toast

Preparation time: 5 minutes
Cooking time: 0 minutes

Servings: 2
Ingredients:

- 2 whole wheat bread slices, toasted
- 1 teaspoon water
- 1 tablespoon tahini paste
- 2 teaspoons feta cheese, crumbled
- Juice of ½ lemon
- 2 teaspoons pine nuts
- A pinch of black pepper

Directions:

1. Combine the tahini, water, and lemon juice in a bowl. Whisk well before spreading the mixture over the toasted bread pieces.
2. Add the remaining ingredients to each dish and serve as breakfast.

Nutrition:

Calories: 142, Fat: 7.6, Carbs: 13.7, Protein: 5.8

Cheesy Olives Bread

Preparation time: 1 hour and 40 minutes
Cooking time: 30 minutes
Servings: 10
Ingredients:

- 4 cups whole-wheat flour
- 3 tablespoons oregano, chopped
- 2 teaspoons dry yeast
- ¼ cup olive oil and
- ½ cups black olives, pitted and sliced
- 1 cup water
- ½ cup feta cheese, crumbled

Directions:

1. In a bowl, combine the flour, water, yeast, and oil. Stir and thoroughly knead the dough. The dough should be placed in a basin, covered with plastic wrap, and kept warm for an hour.

2. Split the dough into two dishes and give each ball a lot of stretching. Each ball should have the remaining ingredients added to it, and each one should have the dough well kneaded.

3. Flatten the balls slightly and set them aside for a further 40 minutes. Place the balls on a parchment-lined baking sheet, slit each one, and bake for 30 minutes at 425 degrees F. As part of a Mediterranean breakfast, serve the bread.

Nutrition:
Calories: 251, Fat: 7.3, Carbs: 39.7, Protein: 6.7

Almonds Crusted Rack of Lamb with Rosemary

Preparation time: 10 minutes
Cooking time: 35 minutes
Servings: 2
Ingredients:

- 1 garlic clove, minced
- ½ tbsp olive oil
- Salt and freshly cracked black pepper
- ¾ lb rack of lamb
- 1 small organic egg
- 1 tbsp breadcrumbs
- 2 oz almonds, finely chopped
- ½ tbsp fresh rosemary, chopped

Directions:
1. Turn on the oven, lower the temperature to 350 degrees, and let the oven to preheat. A baking sheet should be taken, greased with oil, and placed away until needed. In a dish, combine the garlic, oil, salt, and freshly cracked black pepper. Rub this mixture all over the rack of lamb. In a bowl, crack the egg, whisk it to combine, and put it

away until needed. In a separate plate, combine the breadcrumbs with the almonds and rosemary.

2. Place the seasoned rack of lamb on the lined baking sheet after dipping it in the egg and coating it well with the almond mixture. Place the rack of lamb in the oven after it has heated up, and cook for 35 minutes, or until it is well done.

3. Remove the rack of lamb from the oven pan when it is finished, place it on a plate, and serve right immediately. Rack of lamb should be chopped into pieces, distributed equally between two heatproof containers, covered, and stored in the refrigerator for up to three days before serving.

4. Reheat the rack of lamb in the microwave just before serving so it is hot.

Nutrition:
Calories: 471, Fat 31.6g, Carbs 8.5g, Protein: 39g

Sweet Potato Tart

Preparation time: 10 minutes
Cooking time: 1 hour and 10 minutes
Servings: 8
Ingredients:

- 2 pounds sweet potatoes, peeled and cubed
- ¼ cup olive oil+ a drizzle
- 7 ounces feta cheese, crumbled
- 1 yellow onion, chopped
- 2 eggs, whisked
- ¼ cup almond milk
- 1 tablespoon herbs de Provence
- A pinch of salt and black pepper
- 6 phyllo sheets
- 1 tablespoon parmesan, grated

Directions:

1. Spread the potatoes out on a baking sheet covered with parchment paper, drizzle with half the oil, salt, and pepper, and roast for 25 minutes at 400 degrees F.

2. In the meanwhile, heat half of the remaining oil in a skillet over medium heat. Add the onion, and cook for 5 minutes. Combine the eggs, milk, feta, herbs, salt, pepper, onion, sweet potatoes, and the remaining oil in a bowl and toss to incorporate. Place the phyllo sheets in the tart pan and sprinkle some oil over them.

3. Pour the sweet potato mixture onto the pan and smooth it out evenly. Add the parmesan and bake for 20 minutes at 350 degrees F with the foil covering. Take off the foil, bake the tart for a further 20 minutes, let it cool, slice it, and serve it for breakfast.

Nutrition:

Calories: 476, Fat: 16.8, Carbs: 68.8, Protein: 13.9

Blueberries Quinoa

Preparation time: 5 minutes

Cooking time: 0 minutes

Servings: 4

Ingredients:

- 2 cups almond milk
- 2 cups quinoa, already cooked
- ½ teaspoon cinnamon powder
- 1 tablespoon honey
- 1 cup blueberries
- ¼ cup walnuts, chopped

Directions:

1. Toss the quinoa in a dish with the milk and the other ingredients, then serve it in smaller bowls for breakfast.

Nutrition:

Calories: 284, Fat: 14.3, Carbs: 15.4, Protein: 4.4

Kale Chickpea Mash

Preparation Time: 15 minutes

Cooking Time: 12 minutes

Servings: 1

Ingredients:

- 1 shallot
- 3 tablespoons garlic
- A bunch of kale
- 1/2 cup boiled chickpea
- 2 tablespoons coconut oil
- Sea salt

Directions:

1. Garlic is added to olive oil
2. On a nonstick skillet, sauté shallot in oil after being chopped.
3. Continue to cook the shallot until it becomes golden.
4. Stir the greens and garlic into the skillet.
5. Stir in the chickpeas, and simmer for six minutes. Stir well after adding the other ingredients.
6. Provide and savour

Nutrition:

Calories: 149 Fat: 8g Carbs: 13g Protein: 4g

Raspberries and Yogurt Smoothie

Preparation time: 5 minutes

Cooking time: 0 minutes

Servings: 2

Ingredients:

- 2 cups raspberries
- ½ cup Greek yogurt
- ½ cup almond milk
- ½ teaspoon vanilla extract

Directions:

1. Blend the yoghurt, milk, vanilla, and raspberries in a blender until smooth. Pour into 2 glasses and serve as breakfast.
Nutrition:
Calories: 245, Fat: 9.5, Carbs: 5.6, Protein: 1.6

Cheesy Eggs in Avocado

Preparation time: 20 minutes
Cooking time: 15 minutes
Servings: 2
Ingredients:
- 1 medium avocado
- 2 organic eggs
- ¼ cup shredded cheddar cheese
- Salt and freshly cracked black pepper
- 1 tbsp olive oil

Directions:
1. Switch on the oven, then set its temperature to 425°F, and allow preheat. Prepare the avocados in the meanwhile by splitting them in half and removing the pit. Add one avocado half to each muffin tray after greasing the tins with oil.
2. Break an egg into each half of the avocado, cover with cheese, and season with salt and freshly ground black pepper.
3. Once the oven has warmed up, put the muffin pans inside and bake for 15 minutes, or until the muffins are done. When ready, remove the muffin pans, place the cooked organic eggs with avocados on a plate, and then serve.
Nutrition:
Calories: 210, Fat 16.6g, Carbs 6.4g, Protein: 10.7g

Stuffed Pita Breads

Preparation time: 5 minutes
Cooking time: 15 minutes

Servings: 4
Ingredients:

- 1 ½ tablespoons olive oil
- 1 tomato, cubed
- 1 garlic clove, minced
- 1 red onion, chopped
- ¼ cup parsley, chopped
- 15 ounces canned fava beans, drained and rinsed
- ¼ cup lemon juice
- Salt and black pepper to the taste
- 4 whole wheat pita bread pockets

Directions:

1. Add the onion to a skillet that has been heated with oil over medium heat, stir, and cook for 5 minutes.
2. Add the other ingredients, mix, and simmer for an additional 10 minutes. Serve this mixture in the pita pockets as breakfast.

Nutrition:
Calories: 382, Fat: 1.8, Carbs: 66, Protein: 28.5

Eggs and Veggies

Preparation Time: 10 minutes
Cooking Time: 10 minutes
Servings: 4
Ingredients:

- 2 tomatoes, chopped
- 2 eggs, beaten
- 1 bell pepper, chopped
- 1 tsp. tomato paste
- ¼ c. water
- 1 tsp. butter
- ½ white onion, diced
- ½ tsp. chili flakes

- ⅓ tsp. sea salt

Directions:

1. In the pan, melt the butter. Give the bell pepper a thorough swirl occasionally while cooking it for 3 minutes over medium heat.

2. Add the chopped onion and sauté for an additional 2 minutes.

3. In a mixing dish, combine the tomatoes and the veggies.

4. Cook over low heat for 5 minutes. Tomato paste and water should be added. Combine all of the ingredients.

5. Combine the beaten eggs, sea salt, and chilli flakes in a mixing dish.

6. Over medium-low heat, cook for 4 minutes while stirring continuously. The centre of the cooked food ought to be runny.

Nutrition: Calories: 67, Fat: 3.4g, Fiber: 1.5g, Carbs: 6.4g, Protein: 3.8g

Chili Scramble

Preparation Time: 10 minutes
Cooking Time: 13 minutes
Servings: 4

Ingredients:

- 3 tomatoes
- 4 eggs
- ¼ tsp. sea salt
- ½ chili pepper, chopped
- 1 tbsp. butter
- 1 c. water, for cooking

Directions:

1. Fill the pan with water. Water is brought to a boil. After that, add the tomatoes and turn the heat off.

2. Soak the tomatoes in boiling water for two to three minutes.

3. After removing the tomatoes from the water, peel them.

4. In a pot, melted the butter. Sauté the chopped chilli pepper for 3 minutes on medium heat.

5. After that, cut the peeled tomatoes and add them to the chilli peppers.

6. With the veggies, cook for 5 minutes at medium-low heat. They should sometimes be stirred.

7. Add eggs, sea salt, and crack after that.

8. Stir the eggs well with a fork, then fry them for 3 minutes over medium heat.

Nutrition: Calories: 105, Fat: 7.4g, Fiber: 1.1g, Carbs: 4g, Protein: 6.4g

Breakfast Shakshuka

Preparation Time: 10 minutes

Cooking Time: 18 minutes

Servings: 4

Ingredients:

- 1 (14½-oz) can of diced tomatoes, drained
- ¼ tsp turmeric
- 1 c. chopped red bell peppers
- 1 c. finely diced potato
- 2 tbsp. extra-virgin olive oil
- 1 c. chopped shallots
- 1 tsp garlic powder
- ¼ tsp paprika
- ¼ tsp ground cardamom
- 4 large eggs
- ¼ c. chopped fresh cilantro

Directions:

1. Set the oven's temperature to 350°F. The shallots should be sautéed in the olive oil for approximately 3 minutes, turning regularly, until fragrant in a nonstick skillet over medium-high heat.

2. Combine the peppers, potatoes, and garlic powder in a mixing bowl. Cook for 10 minutes with the lid off, stirring every 2 minutes.
3. Combine the tomatoes, cardamom, paprika, turmeric, and in a mixing basin. After it boils, turn off the heat and break the eggs into the pan with the yolks facing up.
4. Put the pan back in the oven for a further 5 to 10 minutes, or until the eggs are cooked to your preference. Serve with cilantro as a garnish.
Nutrition: Calories: 224, Fat: 12g, Carbs: 20g, Protein: 9g

Almond & Maple Quick Grits

Preparation Time: 5 minutes
Cooking Time: 6 minutes
Servings: 4
Ingredients:
- 1½ c. water
- ½ c. unsweetened almond milk
- Pinch of sea salt
- ½ c. quick-cooking grits
- ½ tsp ground cinnamon
- ¼ c. pure maple syrup
- ¼ c. slivered almonds

Directions:
1. Sea salt, water, and almond milk are brought to a boil in a medium saucepan over medium-high heat.
2. While incorporating the grits gradually, stir continuously with a wooden spoon. To avoid lumps, stir the ingredients before slowly bringing it to a boil.
3. Lower the heat to medium-low and stir constantly for a further 5 to 6 minutes, or until all of the water has been absorbed.
4. In a mixing dish, combine the cinnamon, syrup, and almonds. Cook for a further minute while stirring continuously.
Nutrition: Calories: 151, Fat: 4g, Carbs: 28g, Protein: 3g

Pear Pancakes

Preparation Time: 10 minutes
Cooking Time: 15 minutes
Servings: 4

Ingredients:
- 2 eggs
- 1 c. pear, peeled & mashed
- 1 tsp cinnamon
- 2 tsp stevia
- 2 c. whole-wheat flour
- 2 tsp baking powder
- 2 tsp vanilla
- Nonstick cooking spray

Directions:
1.   Beat the eggs in the bowl until they are frothy. Add the flour, pear, baking powder, cinnamon, vanilla, stevia, and continue to whisk just until combined.
2. Spray nonstick cooking spray over the mixture before adding enough batter to the heated pan.
3. Fry the pancakes until the edges are fluffy and dry. Cook until golden on the other side. If preferred, top the pancakes with more pears before serving.

Nutrition: Calories: 174, Fat: 2g, Carbs: 34g, Protein: 5g

Tomato & Zucchini Frittata

Preparation Time: 10 minutes
Cooking Time: 18 minutes
Servings: 4

Ingredients:
- 3 eggs
- 3 egg whites
- ½ c. unsweetened almond milk
- ½ tsp sea salt

- ⅛ tsp freshly ground black pepper
- 2 tbsp. extra-virgin olive oil
- 1 zucchini, chopped
- 8 cherry tomatoes, halved
- ¼ (about 2 oz) c. grated Parmesan cheese

Directions:

1.   In a small mixing dish, combine the eggs, egg whites, almond milk, sea salt, and pepper. Set aside.

2. In a 12-inch oven-safe skillet set over medium-high heat, warm the olive oil. Cook the tomatoes and courgette for 5 minutes, stirring constantly.

3. Simmer the egg mixture for 4 minutes while stirring periodically.

4. With a silicone spatula, remove the set eggs from the pan's edges. By tilting the pan in all directions, let the unset eggs fill in the spaces around the edges.

5. Continue cooking for a further 4 minutes, without stirring, or the edges will curl back.

6. Simmer for 3 to 5 minutes, stirring regularly, or until the cheese melts and the eggs scramble. To serve, cut into wedges.

Nutrition: 223 calories. Carbohydrates: 13g, Protein: 14g, Fat: 4g20.

Blueberry & Vanilla Scones

Preparation Time: 10 minutes
Cooking Time: 10 minutes
Servings: 12 scones

Ingredients:

- 1½ c. almond flour
- 3 organic beaten eggs
- 2 tsp baking powder
- ½ c. stevia
- 2 tsp vanilla extract, unsweetened
- ¾ c. fresh raspberries

- 1 tbsp. olive oil

Directions:

1. Oven temperature set at 375 °F.

2. In a large bowl, whisk together the flour and eggs, add the baking powder, stevia, and vanilla, and toss in the berries until well blended.

3. Use an ice cream scoop to dispense the prepared batter onto a baking dish, spray it with oil, and bake it for 10 minutes or until it is fully cooked.

4. After baking, place the scones on a wire rack to cool thoroughly before serving.

Nutrition: Calories: 133, Fat: 8g, Carbs: 4g, Protein: 2g

Lunch

Spicy, Yogurt-Marinated Chicken Skewers

Preparation Time: 10 minutes
Cooking Time: 12 minutes
Servings: 4-6

Ingredients:

- 1 1/2 tbsp. Aleppo pepper (extra for garnish)
- 3 tsp. crushed garlic
- 1 tsp. freshly ground black pepper
- 2 tsp. Himalayan salt
- 2 tbsp. tomato paste
- 2 tbsp. balsamic vinegar
- 3 tbsp. extra-virgin olive oil (extra for brushing)
- 1 cup plain Greek yogurt
- 1 3/4 lbs. boneless chicken breasts, skins removed, cubed
- 2 unpeeled lemons, thinly sliced (divided)

Directions:

1. Combine the Aleppo pepper with 1 tablespoon of warm water in a large mixing basin, and let aside for 5 minutes, or until the mixture thickens. In a mixing dish, combine the yoghurt, tomato paste, vinegar, olive oil, garlic, pepper, and salt. In a mixing dish, combine the chicken cubes and half of the lemon segments. Toss everything together to coat. Place the bowl in the refrigerator for at least an hour and then cover with plastic wrap.

2. Soak 10 to 12 wooden skewers in a dish of water for 20 minutes to prevent charring.

3. Light a grill, add more olive oil, and set the temperature to medium-high. while the grill is prepared and heated. Reserving the marinade, thread the marinated chicken cubes onto the wet skewers. Cook the skewers on the grill for 10 to 12 minutes, rotating them every so often, or until the chicken is well cooked and evenly browned on both sides.

4. Immediately serve the skewers on top of a bed of lemon wedges.
Nutrition:
Calories: 301; Fat: 11g; Carbs: 7g; Protein: 44g

Shrimp Quinoa Bowl With Black Olives
Preparation Time: 10 minutes
Cooking Time: 20 Minutes
Servings: 4
Ingredients:

- 10 black olives, pitted and halved
- ¼ cup olive oil
- 1 cup quinoa
- 1 lemon, cut in wedges
- 1 lb shrimp, peeled and cooked
- 2 tomatoes, sliced
- 2 bell peppers, thinly sliced
- 1 red onion, chopped
- 1 tsp dried dill
- 1 tbsp fresh parsley, chopped
- Salt and black pepper to taste

Directions:
1. In a saucepan over medium heat, add the quinoa and 2 cups of water. Once the food is soft, bring to a boil, then lower the heat and simmer for 12 to 15 minutes.
2. Take it off the fire and fluff with a fork. Olive oil, dill, parsley, salt, and black pepper should all be combined with the quinoa. Add tomatoes, bell peppers, olives, and onion after stirring. Serve topped with lemon wedges and prawn.
Nutrition:
Calories: 662; Fat: 21g; Protein: 79g; Carbs: 38g.

Stir-Fried Chicken & Barley

Preparation Time: 10 minutes

Cooking Time: 15 minutes

Servings: 4

Ingredients:

- 2 cups water
- 1 cup raw quick-cooking barley
- 3 tsp. avocado oil
- 1 lb. boneless chicken breasts, skins removed, cubed
- 1 medium shallot, chopped
- 1/3 tsp. cayenne pepper
- 1/4 tsp. white pepper
- 1/4 tsp. Himalayan salt
- 1/2 tsp. dried basil, crushed
- 1 tsp. dried oregano, crushed
- 2 tsp. crushed garlic
- 2 medium zucchinis, chopped
- 1 tbsp. fresh flat-leaf parsley, chopped
- 1/4 cup Kalamata olives, pitted and halved
- 2 heirloom tomatoes, chopped

Directions:

1. Bring 2 cups of water to a boil over medium heat. Reduce the heat to medium-low after the water begins to boil, then mix in the uncooked barley. Turning the barley occasionally, cook for 10 to 12 minutes with the lid on, or until it is soft. The saucepan should be taken from the heat and let to cool for five minutes.

2. Heat 2 tablespoons of oil in a large frying pan over medium heat while cooking the chicken cubes until they are cooked through. To keep the heat within, transfer to a bowl and cover with foil.

3. In the same pan, let 1 teaspoon of oil heat. The shallots should be added to the hot oil and cooked for about 3 minutes, or until tender. Stir in the cayenne, white pepper, salt, basil, oregano, garlic, and zucchini for a few minutes, or until the zucchini softens.

4. In a mixing dish, combine the parsley, olives, tomatoes, and chicken. Serve over a bed of boiling barley.
Nutrition:
Calories: 403; Fat: 12g; Carbs: 44g; Protein: 31g

Greek-Style Chicken Couscous
Preparation Time: 10 minutes
Cooking Time: 3-4 hours
Servings: 6
Ingredients:
- 1 tbsp. extra-virgin olive oil (plus 1 tsp.)
- 1/2 cup shallots, chopped
- 3 tbsp. crushed garlic
- 6 boneless chicken breast halves, skins removed
- 1 tsp. dried oregano
- 2 tsp. finely grated lemon zest
- 1 tbsp. quick cooking tapioca
- 3 tbsp. sun-dried tomatoes, chopped
- 1/4 cup Kalamata olives, pitted and chopped
- 2 1/2 cups chicken stock (divided)
- 1 3/4 cups raw couscous
- 1/2 cup crumbled feta cheese

Directions:
1. Heat 1 tablespoon of oil in a small frying pan over medium heat before adding the shallots and cooking for 3 minutes, or until the shallots become transparent. Add the garlic, stir, and cook for another minute.
2. Add the chicken, oregano, zest, tapioca, tomatoes, olives, shallots, and 3/4 cup chicken stock to a large slow cooker. On the lowest heat setting, cook the chicken for 3–4 hours, or until it is well cooked. Chicken may be diced or shredded as desired. The chicken may also be prepared whole.

3. Bring the remaining stock and olive oil to a boil in a big pot over medium heat. Add the uncooked couscous to the pot after transferring it to a stable chopping board. 5 minutes should pass for the couscous to stand, or until the liquid has entirely absorbed.
4. Top the couscous with feta cheese and serve the grilled chicken.
Nutrition:
Calories: 475; Fat: 11g; Carbs: 48g; Protein: 44g

Pan-fried Chili Sea Scallops
Preparation Time: 10 minutes
Cooking Time: 25 Minutes
Servings: 4
Ingredients:
- 1 ½ lb large sea scallops, tendons removed
- 3 tbsp olive oil
- 1 garlic clove, finely chopped
- ½ red pepper flakes
- 2 tbsp chili sauce
- ¼ cup tomato sauce
- 1 small shallot, minced
- 1 tbsp minced fresh cilantro
- Salt and black pepper to taste

Directions:
1. In a pan over medium heat, warm the olive oil. Scallops should be added and cooked for two minutes without being moved. They should be golden brown and cooked for a further 2 minutes without being moved. Set aside. The shallot and garlic should be added to the pan and cooked for 3 to 5 minutes, or until tender. Stir for 3–4 minutes after adding the chilli sauce, tomato sauce, and red pepper flakes. Re-add the scallops and reheat completely. Add cilantro on top after adjusting the flavour.
Nutrition:

Calories: 204; Fat: 14.1g; Protein: 14g; Carbs: 5g.

Ground Turkey Mince
Preparation Time: 10 minutes
Cooking Time: 10-15 minutes
Servings: 4
Ingredients:
- 2 tbsp. avocado oil
- 1 lb. lean ground turkey
- 2 tsp. crushed garlic
- 1 medium red bell pepper, seeded and diced
- 1 small shallot, chopped
- 1/2 tsp. ground cumin
- 1/2 tsp. ground cinnamon
- Freshly ground black pepper
- 1/4 tsp. kosher salt
- 2 tbsp. hummus
- 1/4 cup chicken bone broth
- 1 lemon, finely zested
- 1 tbsp. lemon juice
- Fresh parsley, chopped, for garnish

Directions:
1. Heat 1 tablespoon of the oil in a large frying pan over medium-high heat. When the oil is hot, add the ground turkey and fry it in one layer, without stirring, for about five minutes. After five minutes, flip the meat over and stir to break up all of the pieces. Scrape into a bowl, then put aside.
2. Reset the heat to medium-low and add the remaining oil to the pan. When the vegetables are tender, fry the shallots, bell peppers, and garlic in the hot oil for about 5 minutes. Before adding the salt, hummus, chicken stock, lemon zest, and lemon juice to the ground

turkey in the pan, stir in the cumin and cinnamon for about 30 seconds. a 5 minute stirring period

3. Place the ground turkey and fresh parsley on your preferred wraps.

Nutrition:

Calories: 280; Fat: 17g; Carbs: 10g; Protein: 23g

Spicy Grilled Shrimp With Lemon Wedges

Preparation Time: 10 minutes

Cooking Time: 6 Minutes

Servings: 6

Ingredients:

- 1 large clove garlic, crushed
- 1 teaspoon coarse salt
- 1 teaspoon paprika
- ½ teaspoon cayenne pepper
- 2 teaspoons lemon juice
- 2 tablespoons plus 1 teaspoon olive oil, divided
- 2 pounds large shrimp, peeled and deveined
- 8 wedges lemon, for garnish

Directions:

1. Turn the grill's heat to medium.

2. In a small bowl, combine the garlic, 2 tablespoons of olive oil, salt, paprika, cayenne pepper, lemon juice, and stir until a paste forms. Add the prawn and stir to thoroughly coat.

3. Lightly brush the remaining 1 teaspoon of olive oil onto the grill grates.

4. Grill the prawn for four to six minutes, turning them over halfway through, or until they are completely opaque and pink.

5. Add lemon wedges as a garnish and serve the shrimp hot.

Nutrition:

Calories: 163; Fat: 5.8g; Protein: 25.2g; Carbs: 2.8g.

Hake Fillet In Herby Tomato Sauce

Preparation Time: 10 minutes
Cooking Time: 30 Minutes
Servings: 4
Ingredients:

- 2 tbsp olive oil
- 1 onion, sliced thin
- 1 fennel bulb, sliced
- Salt and black pepper to taste
- 4 garlic cloves, minced
- 1 tsp fresh thyme, chopped
- 1 can diced tomatoes,
- ½ cup dry white wine
- 4 skinless hake fillets
- 2 tbsp fresh basil, chopped

Directions:

1. In a pan over medium heat, warm the olive oil. The onion and fennel should be softened after 5 minutes of sautéing. Around 30 seconds later, add the garlic and thyme and stir until fragrant. Wine and tomatoes should be added, then simmered.

2. Use salt and pepper to season the hake. Place the hake in the tomato sauce, skin side down, and ladle some sauce on top. reheat to a simmer. Cook hake for 10 to 12 minutes, or until it flakes easily with a fork. Basil should be added before serving.

Nutrition:

Calories: 452; Fat: 9.9g; Protein: 78g; Carbs: 9.7g.

Roasted Red Snapper With Citrus Topping

Preparation Time: 10 minutes
Cooking Time: 35 Minutes
Servings: 2
Ingredients:

- 2 tbsp olive oil
- 1 tsp fresh cilantro, chopped
- ½ tsp grated lemon zest
- ½ tbsp lemon juice
- ½ tsp grated grapefruit zest
- ½ tbsp grapefruit juice
- ½ tsp grated orange zest
- ½ tbsp orange juice
- ½ shallot, minced
- ¼ tsp red pepper flakes
- Salt and black pepper to taste
- 1 whole red snapper, cleaned

Directions:

1. Set the oven to 380 F. In a bowl, combine the olive oil, cilantro, shallot, lemon, orange, and grapefruit juices, as well as the pepper flakes. Add salt and pepper to taste. Before serving, set the citrus topping aside.

2. Combine the lemon, orange, grapefruit, and salt and pepper in a another bowl. Make 3–4 shallow cuts on each side of the snapper with a sharp knife, spaced 2 inches apart. Place the fish on a prepared baking sheet after spooning the citrus mixture into the cavity of the fish. Roast the fish for 25 minutes or until it flakes. Serve with a citrus garnish poured on top and enjoy!

Nutrition:

Calories: 257; Fat: 21g; Protein: 16g; Carbs: 1.6g.

Bell Pepper & Scallop Skillet

Preparation Time: 10 minutes
Cooking Time: 25 Minutes
Servings: 4
Ingredients:

- 3 tbsp olive oil

- 2 celery stalks, sliced
- 2 lb sea scallops, halved
- 3 garlic cloves, minced
- Juice of 1 lime
- 1 red bell pepper, chopped
- 1 tbsp capers, chopped
- 1 tbsp mayonnaise
- 1 tbsp rosemary, chopped
- 1 cup chicken stock

Directions:

1. Warm olive oil in a skillet over medium heat and cook celery and garlic for 2 minutes. Stir in bell pepper, lime juice, capers, rosemary, and stock and bring to a boil. Simmer for 8 minutes. Mix in scallops and mayonnaise and cook for 5 minutes.

Nutrition:

Calories: 310; Fat: 16g; Protein: 9g; Carbs: 33g.

Crispy Herb Crusted Halibut

Preparation Time: 10 minutes
Cooking Time: 20 Minutes
Servings: 4

Ingredients:

- 4 halibut fillets, patted dry
- Extra-virgin olive oil, for brushing
- ½ cup coarsely ground unsalted pistachios
- 1 tablespoon chopped fresh parsley
- 1 teaspoon chopped fresh basil
- 1 teaspoon chopped fresh thyme
- Pinch sea salt
- Pinch freshly ground black pepper

Directions:

1. Set the oven's temperature to 350°F. Use parchment paper to cover a baking sheet.
2. Arrange the fillets on the baking sheet, then liberally spray them with olive oil.
3. Combine the pistachios, parsley, basil, thyme, salt, and pepper in a small bowl.
4. Distribute the nut mixture evenly over the fish, covering the tops of the fillets.
5. Bake for approximately 20 minutes in the preheated oven, or until it flakes when tested with a fork.
6. Serve right away.

Nutrition:
Calories: 262; Fat: 11.0g; Protein: 32.0g; Carbs: 4.0g.

Curried Duck & Winter Vegetables

Preparation Time: 10 minutes
Cooking Time: 1-2 hours
Servings: 4

Ingredients:
- 1 lb. duck legs or drumsticks
- 1 tsp. crushed garlic
- Himalayan salt
- Freshly ground black pepper
- 1/8 tsp. ground cardamom
- 1/8 tsp. red pepper flakes
- 1/4 tsp. ground turmeric powder
- 1/4 tsp. sweet smoked paprika
- 1/4 tsp. ground cilantro seeds
- 1/4 tsp. ground cumin
- 1/4 tsp. ground ginger
- 3 tbsp. extra-virgin olive oil
- 5.3 oz. chopped cavolo Nero kale, stems removed

- 3 cups Brussels sprouts, halved and trimmed

Directions:

1. Set the wire rack in the centre of the oven and preheat it to 355°F.

2. Lay the duck legs on a wooden cutting board and use a sharp paring knife to create a series of small cuts in the skin and fat. Season the duck liberally with salt and pepper after massaging the garlic into it. The seasoned duck legs should be combined in a large mixing bowl.

3. In a little glass bowl, combine the cardamom, red pepper flakes, turmeric, smoked paprika, cilantro seeds, cumin, and ginger. Duck legs should be coated with the spice mixture. Put the duck legs that have been coated on a baking pan and top with olive oil. halfway through the cooking time, turn the legs over in the oven for one hour and ten minutes.

4. Transfer the cooked duck legs to a serving platter and keep them warm.

5. After the greens and Brussels sprouts are well coated, stir in the rendered duck fat. For another 15 to 20 minutes, or when the vegetables are tender but still crisp, re-bake the baking pan.

6. Place the roasted duck legs next to the prepared vegetables on a serving platter.

Nutrition:

Calories: 658; Fat: 56.6g; Carbs: 8.6g; Protein: 27.3g

Lemon Rosemary Roasted Branzino

Preparation Time: 10 minutes

Cooking Time: 30 Minutes

Servings: 2

Ingredients:

- 4 tablespoons extra-virgin olive oil, divided
- 2 branzino fillets, preferably at least 1 inch thick
- 1 garlic clove, minced
- 1 bunch scallions (white part only), thinly sliced

- 10 to 12 small cherry tomatoes, halved
- 1 large carrot, cut into ¼-inch rounds
- ½ cup dry white wine
- 2 tablespoons paprika
- 2 teaspoons kosher salt
- ½ tablespoon ground chili pepper
- 2 rosemary sprigs or 1 tablespoon dried rosemary
- 1 small lemon, thinly sliced
- ½ cup sliced pitted kalamata olives

Directions:

1. For approximately two minutes, heat a large ovenproof skillet over high heat until hot. When it shimmers, add 1 tablespoon of olive oil and heat for 10 to 15 seconds.

2. Add the branzino fillets and fry for 2 minutes with the skin side up. The fillets should cook for a further 2 minutes after flipping. Set aside.

3. To uniformly coat the pan, swirl 2 tablespoons of olive oil around it.

4. Include the carrot, tomatoes, scallions, garlic, and sauté for 5 minutes or until the carrot is tender.

5. Add the wine and whisk everything together well. Place the fish over the sauce with care.

6. Turn the oven on to 450°F.

7. Season the fillets with paprika, salt, and chilli powder before brushing them with the remaining 1 tablespoon of olive oil. Lemon slices and a rosemary sprig are placed on top of each fillet. Place the fish in the skillet and surround it with the olives.

8. Roast the lemon slices for about 10 minutes, or until they are browned. Serve warm.

Nutrition:

Calories: 524; Fat: 43.0g; Protein: 57.7g; Carbs: 25.0g.

Tuna Gyros With Tzatziki

Preparation Time: 10 minutes
Cooking Time: 15 Minutes
Servings: 4

Ingredients:

- 4 oz tzatziki
- ½ lb canned tuna, drained
- ½ cup tahini
- 4 sundried tomatoes, diced
- 2 tbsp warm water
- 2 garlic cloves, minced
- 1 tbsp lemon juice
- 4 pita wraps
- 5 black olives, chopped
- Salt and black pepper to taste

Directions:

1. Combine the tahini, water, lemon juice, garlic, salt, and black pepper in a bowl. Pita wraps should be warmed in a grill pan for a few minutes while being turned once. Top the tuna, sundried tomatoes, and olives with the tahini and tzatziki sauces that have been spread over the warmed pitas. Slice in half, then serve right away.

Nutrition:

Calories: 334; Fat: 24g; Protein: 21.3g; Carbs: 9g.

Herb-Marinated Chicken & Radish Salad

Preparation Time: 10 minutes
Cooking Time: 50 minutes
Servings: 4

Ingredients:

- 4 boneless chicken breast halves, skins removed
- Himalayan salt

- Freshly ground black pepper
- 2/3 cup Moroccan chermoula
- 1 cup fresh parsley leaves, chopped
- 1/4 red onion, thinly sliced
- 1 English cucumber, thinly sliced
- 12 small radishes, thinly sliced
- 2 tbsp. extra-virgin olive oil
- 1 tbsp. freshly squeezed lemon juice
- 1 tbsp. lightly toasted sesame seeds

Directions:
1. Lay the chicken breasts out on a wooden cutting board, and use a sharp knife to cut a few small slits into each one. Season the breasts well with salt and pepper before placing them in a basin. Put the chermoula over the chicken breasts and chill them for at least an hour or overnight.
2. Set the wire rack in the centre of the oven and preheat it to 400°F.
3. In a baking dish, combine the marinated chicken and marinade. Bake for 45 to 50 minutes, or until the chicken is well cooked. Let the chicken to sit on the counter while you prepare the salad.
4. Combine the radishes, cucumber, onion, and parsley in a large mixing bowl. After the ingredients are well coated, add the olive oil, lemon juice, and 1/4 teaspoon each of salt and pepper.
5. Just before serving, sprinkle the chicken with sesame seeds and place it over a bed of radish salad.

Nutrition:
Calories: 426; Fat: 30g; Carbs: 7g; Protein: 35g

Seafood Stew
Preparation Time: 10 minutes
Cooking Time: 25 Minutes
Servings: 4
Ingredients:
- ½ lb skinless trout, cubed

- 2 tbsp olive oil
- ½ lb clams
- ½ lb cod, cubed
- 1 onion, chopped
- ½ fennel bulb, chopped
- 2 garlic cloves, minced
- ¼ cup dry white wine
- 2 tbsp chopped fresh parsley
- 1 can tomato sauce
- 1 cup fish broth
- 1 tbsp Italian seasoning
- ⅛ tsp red pepper flakes
- Salt and black pepper to taste

Directions:

1. Saute onion and fennel in olive oil for 5 minutes over medium heat. Cook the garlic for 30 seconds after adding it. Cook for one minute after adding the wine. Add tomato sauce, clams, broth, cod, trout, salt, pepper, and Italian seasoning. Stir to combine. Just bring to a boil, then simmer for five minutes. Throw away any unopened clams. Add parsley on top.

Nutrition:

Calories: 372; Fat: 15g; Protein: 34g; Carbs: 25g.

Curried Chicken Patties

Preparation Time: 10 minutes
Cooking Time: 15-20 minutes
Servings: 4

Ingredients:

- 1/3 tsp. freshly ground black pepper
- 1/4 tsp. kosher salt
- 1/2 tsp. ground turmeric powder
- 1 tsp. ground ginger

- 1 tsp. crushed garlic
- 1/4 cup shallots, finely chopped
- 1 lb. ground chicken
- 1 tbsp. avocado oil (more if needed)

Directions:

1. Combine the chicken, pepper, salt, turmeric, ginger, garlic, and shallots in a large mixing bowl. Stir well to combine. Make the chicken into 8 equal-sized patties.

2. In a large frying pan over medium heat, warm one tablespoon of avocado oil. After the oil is hot, fry the patties in batches. Cook the patties for two to three minutes on each side, or until well-browned. Between batches , top out the pan with oil as necessary.

3. Place the heated patties on the buns of your choice.

Nutrition:

Calories: 206; Fat: 14g; Carbs: 1g; Protein: 20g

Veggie & Clam Stew With Chickpeas

Preparation Time: 10 minutes
Cooking Time: 40 Minutes
Servings: 4

Ingredients:

- 2 tbsp olive oil
- 1 yellow onion, chopped
- 1 fennel bulb, chopped
- 1 carrot, chopped
- 1 red bell pepper, chopped
- 2 garlic cloves, minced
- 3 tbsp tomato paste
- 16 oz canned chickpeas, drained
- 1 tsp dried thyme
- ¼ tsp smoked paprika
- Salt and black pepper to taste

- 1 lb clams, scrubbed

Directions:

1. In a saucepan with medium heat, warm the olive oil, then sauté the fennel, onion, bell pepper, and carrot for 5 minutes, or until they are soft. Cook for a further minute after adding the tomato paste and garlic. 2 cups of water, the chickpeas, thyme, paprika, salt, and pepper should all be combined before coming to a boil and cooking for 20 minutes.

2. Run cold, running water over the clams to rinse them. Clams that stay open after being tapped with your fingertips should be discarded. The unopened clams should be added to the saucepan and cooked for 4-5 minutes or until the shells open. Once cooking is complete, throw away any clams that didn't completely open. Add salt and pepper to taste to taste the seasoning. Serve.

Nutrition:

Calories: 460; Fat: 13g; Protein: 35g; Carbs: 48g.

Baked Fish With Pistachio Crust

Preparation Time: 10 minutes
Cooking Time: 15 To 20 Minutes
Servings: 4

Ingredients:

- ½ cup extra-virgin olive oil, divided
- 1 pound flaky white fish (such as cod, haddock, or halibut), skin removed
- ½ cup shelled finely chopped pistachios
- ½ cup ground flaxseed
- Zest and juice of 1 lemon, divided
- 1 teaspoon ground cumin
- 1 teaspoon ground allspice
- ½ teaspoon salt
- ¼ teaspoon freshly ground black pepper

Directions:
1. Set the oven to 400 degrees.
2. Place two teaspoons of olive oil on a baking sheet that has been lined with parchment paper or aluminium foil and spread it out to cover the bottom completely.
3. Separate the fish into four equal pieces and set them on the baking sheet that has been prepared.
4. Mix the pistachios, flaxseed, lemon zest, cumin, allspice, salt, and pepper in a small bowl. Add 1/4 cup of olive oil and mix well.
5. Evenly distribute the nut mixture over the chunks of fish. Depending on the thickness of the fish, bake for 15 to 20 minutes, then drizzle the remaining 2 tablespoons of olive oil and lemon juice over the fish.
5. Let cool completely before serving.

Nutrition:
Calories: 509; Fat: 41.0g; Protein: 26.0g; Carbs: 9.0g.

Dinner

One-Pan Chicken Pecan Bake

Preparation Time: 10 minutes
Cooking Time: 30-60 minutes
Servings: 4
Ingredients:

- 4 whole garlic cloves
- 1/2 medium shallot, diced
- 1 medium green bell pepper, seeded and diced
- 1 medium red bell pepper, seeded and diced
- 2 lbs. chicken drumsticks
- 2 tbsp. avocado oil
- Freshly ground black pepper
- 1/2 tsp. kosher salt
- 1 tsp. dried basil
- 1 tsp. dried thyme
- 1/2 cup pecan halves
- 2 tbsp. red wine vinegar

Directions:

1. Wrap a large, rimmed baking pan with greaseproof paper, and then preheat the oven to 400°F. Position a wire rack in the centre of the oven.

2. Place the drumsticks, garlic, shallots, bell peppers, and them in a single layer in the prepared baking pan.

3. Cover everything with the oil. Black pepper, salt, basil, and thyme should all be thoroughly sprinkled over the pan's contents. Add some pecans to the mixture.

4. Set the oven to 350 degrees Fahrenheit and preheat it for 30 minutes, flipping the chicken and tossing the vegetables halfway through. When the vegetables are tender yet crisp and the

drumsticks are wonderfully browned, take the pan out of the oven and add the vinegar. Add the vinegar and serve right away.

Nutrition:

Calories: 391; Fat: 28g; Carbs: 11g; Protein: 27g

Ouzo & Orange Glazed Duck

Preparation Time: 10 minutes

Cooking Time: 15 minutes

Servings: 4

Ingredients:

- 2 duck breast halves
- 1 tsp. flaky sea salt (plus a pinch)
- 1 tbsp. extra-virgin olive oil
- 1/2 cup fennel bulbs, chopped (fronds reserved for topping)
- 1 bird's eye chili, halved and seeded
- 1 small red onion, diced
- 1/4 cup ouzo
- 1/2 cup freshly squeezed orange juice
- 1 cup chicken stock
- Freshly ground black pepper

Directions:

1. Arrange the duck breast halves on a strong cutting board, skin side up. Using a sharp paring knife, make a large X across each breast, cutting through the skin and fat but avoiding the meat. The breasts should be salted, then set aside for five minutes.

2. In a big pot over medium heat, warm the olive oil. Place the breasts skin side down in the pan once the oil is hot and sear for 8–10 minutes. Using tongs, turn the breasts over, then sear the bottom halves for an additional 3 minutes. The seared breasts should be transferred to a bowl and left to remain warm. As the rest of the dinner is being made, they should sit for about 10 minutes.

3. In the meanwhile, sauté the fennel bulbs, chile, and onion in the same pan for about 3 minutes, or until the vegetables soften. Pour the ouzo into the pan while it is on a wooden cutting board. To prevent catching fire at this phase, take additional precautions. To remove any food that has stuck to the bottom, put the pan back on the heat and stir the contents with a wooden spoon. You should use half as much ouzo.

4. Add a little more salt and then add the orange juice and stock. Stirring periodically, let the sauce boil for 5 minutes or until it is thick enough to coat the back of a wooden spoon. Get rid of the heat.

5. Working against the grain, slice the duck breasts into 1/8-inch-thick slices. Plate the slices while they are still warm, then garnish with the sauce and fennel fronds.

Nutrition:
Calories: 229; Fat: 9g; Carbs: 7g; Protein: 27g

One-skillet Salmon With Olives & Escarole

Preparation Time: 10 minutes
Cooking Time: 25 Minutes
Servings: 4

Ingredients:
- 3 tbsp olive oil
- 1 head escarole, torn
- 4 salmon fillets, boneless
- 1 lime, juiced
- Salt and black pepper to taste
- ¼ cup fish stock
- ¼ cup green olives, pitted and chopped
- ¼ cup fresh chives, chopped

Directions:
1. In a medium-sized pan, heat the remaining olive oil, add the escarole, lime juice, salt, pepper, fish stock, and olives, and cook for 6 minutes. Divide among plates. In the same skillet, preheat the

remaining oil. Add salt and pepper to the salmon, then cook it for 8 minutes on each side, or until golden brown. Serve heated, topped with chives, on the escarole plates.

Nutrition:

Calories: 280; Fat: 15g; Protein: 19g; Carbs: 25g.

Lemon-Simmered Chicken & Artichokes

Preparation Time: 10 minutes

Cooking Time: 10-15 minutes

Servings: 4

Ingredients:

- 4 boneless chicken breast halves, skins removed
- 1/4 tsp. Himalayan salt
- 1/4 tsp. freshly ground black pepper
- 2 tsp. avocado oil
- 1 tbsp. lemon juice
- 2 tsp. dried crushed oregano
- 1/4 cup Kalamata olives, pitted and halved
- 2/3 cup reduced-sodium chicken stock
- 14 oz. canned, water-packed, quartered artichoke hearts

Directions:

1. Add salt and pepper to taste and season the chicken breasts. In a big pan, heat the oil on medium-high. In heated oil, brown the chicken for two to four minutes on each side.

2. After the chicken is beautifully browned, add the artichoke hearts, oregano, lemon juice, and olives. After the liquid has boiled, reduce the heat to low, cover the pan, and let the chicken simmer for 4-5 minutes more.

3. Serve immediately.

Nutrition:

Calories: 225; Fat: 9g; Carbs: 9g; Protein: 26g

Spiced Flounder With Pasta Salad

Preparation Time: 10 minutes
Cooking Time: 25 Minutes
Servings: 4

Ingredients:

- 2 tbsp olive oil
- 4 flounder fillets, boneless
- 1 tsp rosemary, dried
- 2 tsp cumin, ground
- 1 tbsp coriander, ground
- 2 tsp cinnamon powder
- 2 tsp oregano, dried
- Salt and black pepper to taste
- 2 cups macaroni, cooked
- 1 cup cherry tomatoes, halved
- 1 avocado, peeled and sliced
- 1 cucumber, cubed
- ½ cup black olives, sliced
- 1 lemon, juiced

Directions:

1. Turn the oven on at 390 °F. In a bowl, mix the oregano, cinnamon, cumin, coriander, rosemary, salt, and pepper. Flake should be added and coated.

2. In a skillet set over medium heat, warm the olive oil. The fish fillets should be browned for 4 minutes on each side. Place on a baking sheet and bake for 7 to 10 minutes. Toss the mac & cheese, tomatoes, avocado, cucumber, olives, and lemon juice together in a bowl. Pasta salad should be served with the fish.

Nutrition:

Calories: 370; Fat: 16g; Protein: 26g; Carbs: 57g.

Curried Chickpea Burgers

Preparation Time: 10 minutes
Cooking Time: 10-15 minutes
Servings: 6

Ingredients:

- 1/4 cup fat-free red wine vinaigrette
- 1 medium shallot, thinly sliced
- 1/4 cup fresh parsley
- 1/4 cup panko breadcrumbs
- 1/3 cup lightly toasted walnuts, chopped
- 15 oz. canned chickpeas, drained and rinsed
- 1/2 tsp. white pepper
- 1 tsp. curry powder
- 1 tsp. ground turmeric
- 2 large free-range eggs
- 2 tbsp. French mustard
- 1/3 cup fat-free mayonnaise
- 6 sesame seed hamburger buns, split and toasted
- 6 romaine lettuce leaves
- 3 tbsp. fresh basil leaves, lightly chopped

Directions:

1. Position the wire rack in the top third of the oven and warm to 375°F. Spray some baking spray on a baking sheet.

2. Put the shallot pieces in a shallow basin with the vinaigrette. Set aside.

3. In a food processor, pulse the parsley, breadcrumbs, walnuts, and chickpeas several times on high speed to thoroughly incorporate the ingredients. Then pulse one more until there are no lumps before adding the pepper, curry powder, turmeric, and eggs.

4. Create six roughly equal-sized patties out of the mixture, and set them on the baking sheet that has been prepared. The patties should be baked for 10 to 15 minutes, or until well done.

5. Combine the mayonnaise and mustard in a little glass bowl. Each bun's open side should have the substance spread over it.
6. Arrange a single lettuce leaf and the wet shallots on top of each bun. Place one cooked patties on each bun, top with basil leaves, then close the burgers. Serve immediately.
Nutrition:
Calories: 386; Fat: 12g; Carbs: 54g; Protein: 16g

Hot Tomato & Caper Squid Stew
Preparation Time: 10 minutes
Cooking Time: 50 Minutes
Servings: 4
Ingredients:
- 1 cans whole peeled tomatoes, diced
- ¼ cup olive oil
- 1 onion, chopped
- 1 celery rib, sliced
- 3 garlic cloves, minced
- ¼ tsp red pepper flakes
- 1 red chili, minced
- ½ cup dry white wine
- 2 lb squid, sliced into rings
- Salt and black pepper to taste
- $^1/_3$ cup green olives, chopped
- 1 tbsp capers
- 2 tbsp fresh parsley, chopped

Directions:
1. In a saucepan set over medium heat, warm the olive oil. For approximately 5 minutes, sauté the onion, garlic, red chile, and celery until they are tender. Pepper flakes are added and cooked for around 30 seconds. Cook for about a minute, scraping off any browned parts as you go, then add the wine. Add a cup of water and

salt and pepper to taste. In the saucepan, stir the squid. Simmer for around 15 minutes, with the heat reduced to low and the lid on, until the squid has released its liquid. Cook the tomatoes, olives, and capers before adding them to the squid. This should take 30-35 minutes. Add parsley on top. Dispense and savour!

Nutrition:
Calories: 334; Fat: 12g; Protein: 28g; Carbs: 30g.

Ricotta Salata Pasta
Preparation Time: 10 minutes
Cooking Time: 15 minutes
Servings: 4
Ingredients:
- 1 lb. fusilli
- 1/3 cup avocado oil
- 1/4 tsp. white pepper
- 1/2 tsp. lemon zest, finely grated
- 1 tbsp. freshly squeezed lemon juice
- 3 tsp. crushed garlic
- 2 cups fresh mint leaves, chopped (more for garnish)
- 1/4 cup almond slivers
- 1/2 cup ricotta Salata, grated (more for garnish)

Directions:
1. Prepare the fusilli in salted water as directed on the box.
2. In the meanwhile, in a food processor, process the avocado oil, pepper, zest, lemon juice, garlic, mint leaves, and almond slivers on high until a lump-free sauce forms. Add 1/2 cup of cheese, and pulse a few times to thoroughly incorporate everything.
3. Once the pasta has finished cooking, strain it through a colander positioned over the washbasin. Scrape the sauce from the food processor over the cooked pasta and transfer to a serving dish. Stir gently to mix. Before serving hot, garnish with additional cheese and mint.

Nutrition:
Calories: 619; Fat: 31g Carbs: 70g; Protein: 21g

Lemon Trout With Roasted Beets

Preparation Time: 10 minutes
Cooking Time: 45 Minutes
Servings: 4
Ingredients:

- 1 lb medium beets, peeled and sliced
- 3 tbsp olive oil
- 4 trout fillets, boneless
- Salt and black pepper to taste
- 1 tbsp rosemary, chopped
- 2 spring onions, chopped
- 2 tbsp lemon juice
- ½ cup vegetable stock

Directions:
1. Set the oven to 390 F. Use parchment paper to cover a baking sheet. The beets should be arranged on the baking pan, salted and peppered, and drizzled with olive oil. For 20 minutes, roast.
2. In a skillet set over medium heat, warm the remaining oil. Trout fillets should be cooked for 8 minutes total, on both sides. Stir in the spring onions and cook for two minutes. Stock and lemon juice should be stirred in after the sauce has been cooking for 5 to 6 minutes. Transfer the beets to a platter, then add the fish fillets on top. Sprinkle rosemary on top after spreading the sauce all over.
Nutrition:
Calories: 240; Fat: 6g; Protein: 18g; Carbs: 22g.

Cauliflower Steaks & Romesco Sauce

Preparation Time: 10 minutes

Cooking Time: 25 minutes
Servings: 4
Ingredients:

- 1 small cauliflower head, stem removed
- White pepper
- Kosher salt
- 1/2 tsp. onion powder
- 1/4 tsp. garlic powder
- extra-virgin avocado oil
- 1 medium red pepper
- 15 oz. canned chickpeas, drained and rinsed
- 1 tsp. freshly squeezed lemon juice
- 1 tsp. crushed garlic
- 1 tbsp. tomato paste
- 1/4 cup almond slivers
- 1/4 cup Greek olives, pitted and sliced
- Fresh parsley, chopped, for garnish

Directions:

1. Line a large baking sheet with greaseproof paper, preheat the oven to 450°F, and place a wire rack in the middle of the oven.

2. Lay the head of cauliflower on a wooden cutting board and cut it into four steaks that are each 1 inch thick. Place the steaks on the baking pan that has been prepared. Combine 1 teaspoon each of pepper, salt, onion powder, and garlic powder in a little glass bowl. Add a teaspoon of olive oil to the top of each steak before seasoning with a few sprinklings of the spice combination. Repeat the technique with another side of the steak, extra olive oil, and any leftover seasoning. Place the entire bell pepper on the tray, and then add 1 teaspoon of oil.

3. Bake the tray in the oven for 15 minutes, or until the skin is browned and the bell pepper is beautifully roasted. Transfer the roasted bell pepper to a paper bag after removing the baking sheet

from the oven. Set aside after folding the sides over to stifle the steam.

4. In a medium bowl, combine the chickpeas, 1 teaspoon of oil, and a good dose of salt and pepper. Coat by tossing. Use a spatula to turn the cauliflower steaks after adding the coated chickpeas to the pan. After the steaks are cooked through and crispy on the exterior, place the dish back in the oven for a further 10 minutes.

5. Remove the hot bell pepper from the bag with caution. Slice, then take out the seeds and stem. Put the slices, lemon juice, garlic, tomato paste, almond slivers, and 1/4 teaspoon of each salt and pepper in a powerful food processor. Once you get a smooth paste, high-speed pulse.

6. Arrange the roasted chickpeas on top of the cauliflower steaks on the plate. Before adding the olives and parsley garnish, drizzle with the romesco sauce. Serve warm.

Nutrition:
Calories: 360; Fat: 25g; Carbs: 29g; Protein: 11g

Crispy Salmon Patties With Grecian Sauce

Preparation Time: 10 minutes
Cooking Time: 30 Minutes
Servings: 2
Ingredients:

- 1 cup tzatziki sauce
- 2 tsp olive oil
- Salmon cakes
- 6 oz cooked salmon, flaked
- ¼ cup celery, minced
- ¼ cup onion, minced
- ¼ tsp chili powder
- ½ tsp dried dill
- 1 tbsp fresh minced parsley

- Salt and black pepper to taste
- 1 egg, beaten
- ½ cup breadcrumbs

Directions:

1. Combine all the salmon cake ingredients in a large bowl. The mixture should be rolled into balls, then pressed to create patties.

2. In a pan over medium heat, warm the olive oil. The patties should be cooked for 3 minutes on each side or until golden brown. Top the salmon cakes with tzatziki sauce before serving.

Nutrition:

Calories: 555; Fat: 41g; Protein: 31g; Carbs: 18g.

Zesty, Lettuce-Wrapped Chicken Gyros

Preparation Time: 10 minutes

Cooking Time: 30 minutes

Servings: 4

Ingredients:

- 1 1/2 lbs. boneless chicken breasts, skins removed
- 1/2 tsp. white pepper
- 1/2 tsp. kosher salt
- 1/2 tsp. dried thyme
- 1/2 tsp. dried oregano
- 1/2 tsp. ground cumin
- 1 tsp. crushed garlic
- 2 tbsp. freshly squeezed lemon juice
- 1 lemon, zested
- 8 outer leaves of romaine lettuce
- Tahini sauce
- 4 thin dill pickle spears
- Very thinly sliced red onion
- 1 heirloom tomato, sliced

Directions:

1. Place the chicken breasts on a wooden cutting board and cover with greaseproof paper. The breasts should be pounded with a wooden mallet to a thickness of about 1/4 inch before being cut into 6 strips.

2. In a large mixing bowl, combine the pepper, salt, thyme, oregano, cumin, garlic, lemon juice, and lemon zest. Add the chicken strips and toss to coat. Place the bowl in the refrigerator for at least 30 minutes after wrapping it with plastic wrap.

3. Once the chicken has sufficiently cooled, preheat the oven's broiler to low. Position the wire rack around six inches away from the broiler. Broil the chicken strips for 7 minutes, or until they are just cooked through, on a baking sheet coated with foil.

4. Place the dill spears, red onions, and tomato slices on top of each lettuce leaf, then top with a generous dollop of tahini sauce. Between the leaves, fold the cooked chicken and serve it.

Nutrition:
Calories: 150; Fat: 3g; Carbs: 2g; Protein: 26g

One-Pot Curried Halloumi

Preparation Time: 10 minutes
Cooking Time: 20-30 minutes
Servings: 4
Ingredients:

- 2 tbsp. extra-virgin olive oil
- 2 packs halloumi cheese
- 1 cup water
- 1/2 cup coconut milk
- 1/4 cup tomato paste
- 1/4 tsp. white pepper
- 1/2 tsp. ground turmeric
- 1 1/2 tsp. mild curry powder
- 1/2 tsp. garlic powder

- 1 tsp. onion powder
- 1 small cauliflower, cut into small florets
- Himalayan salt
- 2 tbsp. coconut flour
- Fresh coriander leaves, chopped, for serving
- Cooked rice for serving

Directions:

1. Heat the olive oil in a large frying pan over medium-high heat. Cut the halloumi into 8 slices that are each approximately 3/4" thick. Add the halloumi to the pan after the oil is good and heated. If all of the cheese does not fit in the pan comfortably, you may work in batches. Halloumi should be fried till golden brown on both sides. If turning the cheese first proves challenging, don't worry; it will become simpler as the outside coating gets crisper. Place on a dish and reheat as needed.

2. Add the water, coconut milk, tomato paste, pepper, turmeric, curry powder, garlic powder, and onion powder to the same frying pan. Add the cauliflower florets and salt to taste after the sauce has started to boil. When the cauliflower is fork-tender, simmer the florets for 7 to 10 minutes with the pan cover on.

3. Add the coconut flour to the pan after the cauliflower is cooked through and stir until the sauce thickens. After heated thoroughly, add the cooked halloumi.

4. Serve the rice of your choice and the curried halloumi on a plate with the sauce. Serve hot and garnish with coriander leaves.

Nutrition:

Calories: 590; Fat: 48.1g; Carbs: 8.8 g; Protein: 29.2 g

Mackerel And Green Bean Salad

Preparation Time: 10 minutes
Cooking Time: 10 Minutes
Servings: 2
Ingredients:

- 2 cups green beans
- 1 tablespoon avocado oil
- 2 mackerel fillets
- 4 cups mixed salad greens
- 2 hard-boiled eggs, sliced
- 1 avocado, sliced
- 2 tablespoons lemon juice
- 2 tablespoons olive oil
- 1 teaspoon Dijon mustard
- Salt and black pepper, to taste

Directions:

1. Boil the green beans for approximately 3 minutes, or until they are crisp-tender, in a medium pot. Drain, then set apart.

2. Over a medium heat, liquefy the avocado oil in the pan. Cook the mackerel fillets for 4 minutes on each side after adding them.

3. Distribute the salad greens between two dishes. Add avocado slices, cut eggs, and mackerel on the top.

4. Combine the lemon juice, olive oil, mustard, salt, and pepper in a separate dish, then sprinkle the mixture over the salad. After adding and combining the cooked green beans, serve.

Nutrition:

Calories: 437; Fat: 57.3g; Protein: 34.2g; Carbs: 22.1g.

Crispy Vegetable Paella

Preparation Time: 10 minutes

Cooking Time: 35 minutes

Servings: 4

Ingredients:

- 3 tbsp. warm water
- 8 threads of fresh saffron
- 3 cups vegetable stock
- 1 tbsp. extra-virgin avocado oil

- 1 large shallot, thinly sliced
- 4 tsp. crushed garlic
- 1 red bell pepper, thinly sliced
- 1 tsp. kosher salt
- 1/2 tsp. freshly ground black pepper
- 2 tbsp. tomato paste
- 3/4 cups canned crushed tomatoes
- 1 1/2 tsp. sweet smoked paprika
- 1 cup uncooked white rice
- 15 oz. canned chickpeas, drained and rinsed
- 1 1/2 cups haricot verts, trimmed and halved
- 1 lime, cut into wedges, for serving

Directions:

1. In a little glass dish, gently whisk the saffron and warm water together. As you prepare the remainder of the meal, let the dish sit on the counter.

2. Over medium-high heat, simmer the vegetable stock in a medium saucepan. Reduce the heat after the stock starts to simmer in order to keep a very soft simmer.

3. In a big frying pan, heat the avocado oil over medium-high heat. The shallots should only be softened and transparent after approximately 5 minutes of frying, so stir them in. Stir for an extra 30 seconds after adding the garlic to let the flavours mingle. Add the peppers and cook for a further 7 minutes, or until they are soft. Stir in the saffron, tomato paste, crushed tomatoes, sweet smoked paprika, salt, and pepper once the saffron has been given time to soak.

4. Add the haricot verts, chickpeas, and uncooked rice to the simmering broth. Medium-high heat should be used to bring the mixture to a boil, then it should be lowered to a simmer for approximately 20 minutes, or until the rice is cooked and the liquid has been reduced.

5. Spoon the hot cooked rice and veggies into bowls and top with lime wedges.
Nutrition:
Calories: 709; Fat: 12g; Carbs: 121g; Protein: 33g

Vegetable & Herb Chicken Cacciatore
Preparation Time: 10 minutes
Cooking Time: 1 hour10 minutes
Servings: 6-8
Ingredients:

- 1 cup boiling water
- 1/2 oz. dried porcini mushrooms
- 2 tbsp. avocado oil
- 12 boneless chicken thighs, skins removed and fat trimmed
- 1 large fennel bulb, cored, halved, and thinly sliced
- 1 large shallot, halved and thinly sliced
- 1 large green bell pepper, seeded, and chopped into rings
- 1 tsp. fresh thyme leaves, chopped
- 2 tsp. finely grated orange zest
- 1 tbsp. fresh rosemary, chopped
- 3 tsp. crushed garlic
- 3 tbsp. balsamic vinegar
- 1 tsp. kosher salt
- 2 tbsp. tomato paste
- 3/4 cup dry white wine

Directions:
1. Set the wire rack in the centre of the oven and preheat it to 350°F.
2. Place the mushrooms and boiling water in a large mixing bowl, and leave for 20 minutes.
3. In the meanwhile, heat the olive oil in a large frying pan over medium-high heat before browning the chicken thighs on both sides. To avoid overcrowding the pan, you may cook the chicken in

batches if required. The cooked chicken thighs should be put in a large casserole dish.

4. Lower the heat to low and add the bell pepper, fennel, and shallots to the same pan. Cook the vegetables for 5 minutes, or until they are soft to the touch. In a mixing bowl, combine the thyme, zest, rosemary, and garlic. After 30 seconds, add the vinegar and cook for a further minute.

5. Finely chop the mushrooms before adding them together with the soaking water, salt, tomato paste, and wine.

6. Gently pour the sauce over the chicken thighs in the casserole dish after it has begun to boil. Bake the dish with foil on for 45 minutes.

7. Before serving the hot thighs, let the cooked thighs rest for 5 to 10 minutes.

Nutrition:
Calories: 468; Fat: 19g; Carbs: 9g; Protein: 58g

Cod Fettuccine

Preparation Time: 10 minutes
Cooking Time: 30 Minutes
Servings: 4
Ingredients:
- 1 lb cod fillets, cubed
- 16 oz fettuccine
- 3 tbsp olive oil
- 1 onion, finely chopped
- Salt and lemon pepper to taste
- 1 ½ cups heavy cream
- 1 cup Parmesan cheese, grated

Directions:
1. In a medium-sized saucepan, bring salted water to a boil before adding the fettuccine. Cook as directed on the box, then drain. In a large saucepan, heat the olive oil over medium heat before adding the onion. until tender, stir-fry for 3 minutes. Cod should be salted

and lemon peppered before being added to a pot. Cook cod for 4-5 minutes, or until it flakes easily when tested with a fork. Add heavy cream, and stir for two minutes. Pasta should be added and carefully mixed in. 3–4 minutes of cooking time is needed to slightly thicken the sauce. Add some Parmesan cheese.

Nutrition:
Calories: 431; Fat: 36g; Protein: 42g; Carbs: 97g.

Fennel Poached Cod With Tomatoes

Preparation Time: 10 minutes
Cooking Time: 20 Minutes
Servings: 4

Ingredients:
- 1 tablespoon olive oil
- 1 cup thinly sliced fennel
- ½ cup thinly sliced onion
- 1 tablespoon minced garlic
- 1 can diced tomatoes
- 2 cups chicken broth
- ½ cup white wine
- Juice and zest of 1 orange
- 1 pinch red pepper flakes
- 1 bay leaf
- 1 pound cod

Directions:
1. In a big skillet, heat up the olive oil. When transparent, add the onion and fennel and simmer for a further 6 minutes, stirring regularly. Cook for another minute after adding the garlic.
2. Stirring the ingredients for 5 minutes, add the tomatoes, chicken broth, wine, orange juice and zest, red pepper flakes, and bay leaf.
3. Gently put the cod in one layer, cover the pot, and boil for 6–7 minutes.

4. Place the fish on a serving platter, top with the remaining sauce, and serve.
Nutrition:
Calories: 336; Fat: 12.5g; Protein: 45.1g; Carbs: 11.0g.

White Bean, Zucchini, & Squash Casserole

Preparation Time: 10 minutes
Cooking Time: 1 hour
Servings: 6
Ingredients:

- 1 small butternut squash
- 1 tsp. freshly ground black pepper
- 1/2 tsp. kosher salt
- 1 tsp. crushed dried oregano
- 1 tsp. crushed garlic
- 1 tbsp. freshly squeezed lemon juice
- 1 tbsp. nutritional yeast
- Extra-virgin olive oil
- 8 oz. canned tomato sauce
- 1/4 medium shallot, diced
- 1 medium zucchini, diced
- 2 cups frozen lima beans, thawed
- 4 oz. Swiss goat cheese, grated
- Fresh coriander leaves for garnish

Directions:
1. Position the wire rack in the middle of the oven and set the oven to 375°F for preheating. Spray some olive oil on a big casserole dish.
2. Make little holes all over the squash skin with a fork. After cutting the squash in half lengthwise, trim the ends. Before heating for one minute on high, take the seeds out. Slice the squash into bite-sized pieces after removing the peel. Put the cubes in a large mixing dish.

3. Stir together the tomato sauce, shallots, zucchini, lima beans, pepper, salt, oregano, garlic, lemon juice, yeast, and 1 teaspoon of olive oil in the bowl.

4. Add the cheese and stir. Scrape the mixture into the casserole dish you just prepared. When the cheese and sauce are bubbling and the veggies are soft to the fork, cover the dish with aluminium foil and bake for 30 to 40 minutes.

5. To serve the casserole hot, sprinkle with the chopped coriander leaves and a few drops of extra virgin olive oil.

Nutrition:

Calories: 176; Fat: 7g; Carbs: 22g; Protein: 9g

Lemon Grilled Shrimp

Preparation Time: 10 minutes
Cooking Time: 4 To 6 Minutes
Servings: 4
Ingredients:

- 2 tablespoons garlic, minced
- 3 tablespoons fresh Italian parsley, finely chopped
- ¼ cup extra-virgin olive oil
- ½ cup lemon juice
- 1 teaspoon salt
- 2 pounds jumbo shrimp, peeled and deveined
- Special Equipment:
- 4 skewers, soaked in water for at least 30 minutes

Directions:

1. In a large bowl, stir the garlic, parsley, olive oil, lemon juice, and salt.

2. Include the shrimp in the dish and mix them well to coat them with the marinade. Set aside for 15 minutes of sitting.

3. When ready, poke a hole in the middle of each prawn with a skewer. On each skewer, you may fit 5 to 6 shrimp.

4. Turn the grill's heat to high.

5. Grill the prawn for 4 to 6 minutes, turning them over halfway through cooking, or until they are opaque in the middle and have a pink exterior.

6. Present hot.

Nutrition:

Calories: 401; Fat: 17.8g; Protein: 56.9g; Carbs: 3.9g.

Italian-Style Slow Cooker Chicken

Preparation Time: 10 minutes

Cooking Time: 5-6 hours

Servings: 6

Ingredients:

- 1 tsp. white pepper
- 1 tsp. kosher salt
- 1/4 tsp. red pepper flakes
- 2 tsp. sweet smoked paprika
- 3 lbs. boneless chicken breast halves, skins removed
- 14 oz. canned, water-packed artichoke hearts, drained and rinsed
- 1 medium shallot, chopped
- 1 sweet red pepper, chopped
- 1/2 lb. button mushrooms, cleaned, and stems removed
- 2 tbsp. fresh thyme leaves, chopped
- 3 tsp. crushed garlic
- 16 oz. canned tomato paste
- 1 1/2 cups chardonnay
- Hot cooked pasta for serving
- Parmesan cheese, grated, for garnish
- 1/4 cup fresh parsley, chopped, for garnish

Directions:

1. In a little glass dish, stir the paprika, pepper, salt, and red pepper flakes. In a large slow cooker, add the chicken breasts and sprinkle

with the spice mixture. Using your hands, spread the spice evenly over the chicken. In a mixing bowl, combine the mushrooms, shallots, sweet red pepper, and artichoke hearts.

2. In a medium-sized mixing bowl, stir the thyme, garlic, tomato paste, and chardonnay until thoroughly combined. Over the slow cooker's ingredients, pour the mixture.

3. After the chicken is done, cover the slow cooker and let it simmer for 5 to 6 hours.

4. Top the spaghetti with warm vegetables and parmesan cheese before serving.

Nutrition:

Calories: 282; Fat: 5g; Carbs: 16g; Protein: 43g

Snacks

Grilled Watermelon

Preparation Time: 10 minutes
Cooking Time: 4 minutes
Servings: 4

Ingredients:

- 1 watermelon, peeled and cut into 1-inch-thick wedges
- 1 garlic clove, minced finely
- 2 tablespoons fresh key lime juice
- Pinch of cayenne powder
- Pinch of sea salt

Directions:

1. Turn the grill's heat to high.
2. Oil the grates of the grill.
3. Arrange the chunks of watermelon on the grill and cook for 2 minutes on each side.
4. In the meanwhile, combine the other ingredients in a dish.
5. Pour the garlic mixture over the watermelon slices before serving.

Nutrition:
Calories: 11 Fat: 0 g Carbs: 2.7 g Protein: 0.2 g

Avocado Gazpacho

Preparation Time: 15 minutes
Cooking Time: 15 minutes
Servings: 6

Ingredients:

- 3 large avocados; peeled, pitted, and chopped
- 1/3 cup fresh cilantro leaves
- 3 cups spring water
- 2 tablespoons fresh key lime juice
- ¼ teaspoon cayenne powder

- Sea salt, as needed

Directions:

1. Combine all ingredients in a powerful blender, and mix until smooth.
2. Spoon the soup into a large bowl.
3. Chill the gazpacho dish in the refrigerator for at least two to three hours before serving.

Nutrition:

Calories: 206 Fat: 4.1 g Carbs: 8.8 g Protein: 1.9 g

Mango Salsa

Preparation Time: 15 minutes

Cooking Time: 15 minutes

Servings: 6

Ingredients:

- 1 avocado; peeled, pitted, and cubed
- 2 tablespoons fresh key lime juice
- 1 mango; peeled, pitted, and cubed
- 1 cup cherry tomatoes, quartered
- 1 tablespoon fresh cilantro, chopped
- Sea salt, as needed

Directions:

1. Combine avocado cubes with lime juice in a bowl.
2. Add the other ingredients to the bowl and mix to incorporate.
3. Serve right away.

Nutrition:

Calories: 108 Fat: 1.4 g Carbs: 12.5 g Protein: 1.4 g

Banana Chips

Preparation Time: 10 minutes

Cooking Time: 1 hour

Servings: 6

Ingredients:
- 5 burro bananas, peeled and cut into ¼-inch-thick slices

Directions:
1. Set the oven to 250°F.
2. Use baking paper to line a large baking sheet.
3. Spread the banana slices out in a single layer on the baking sheet that has been prepared.
4. Bake for around one hour.

Nutrition:
Calories: 88 Fat: 0.1 g Carbs: 22.5 g Protein: 1.1 g

Chickpeas Fries

Preparation Time: 20 minutes
Cooking Time: 50 minutes
Servings: 8

Ingredients:
- 4 cups spring water
- 2 cups chickpea flour
- ½ cup green bell peppers, seeded and chopped
- ½ cup onions, chopped
- 1 tablespoon fresh oregano, chopped
- 1 teaspoon onion powder
- 1 teaspoon cayenne powder
- Sea salt, as needed

Directions:
1. Use oiled parchment paper to cover a baking sheet.
2. Mix the water and flour in a large pan over medium heat until well incorporated.
3. Add the other ingredients and whisk continuously for 10 minutes.
4. Take the mixture from the heat and spread it out on the prepared baking sheet.
5. Smooth the top surface using a spatula.

6. Cover the area with more parchment paper that has been gently oiled, and then firmly press it with a different baking sheet.

7. Let to freeze for 20 minutes.

8. Set the oven to 400°F.

9. Grease a baking sheet very lightly.

10. Take the parchment paper from the top and cut the fries into the appropriate size.

11. Spread the fries out in a single layer on the baking sheet that has been prepared.

12. 20 minutes is about right for baking.

13. Gently turn the fries over, then bake for 10 to 15 minutes.

14. Warm up the food.

Nutrition:

Calories: 98 Fat: 0.2 g Carbs: 15.3 g Protein: 5.4 g

Chilled Mango Treat

Preparation Time: 10 minutes

Cooking Time: 10 minutes

Servings: 4

Ingredients:

- 3 cups frozen mango; peeled, pitted, and chopped
- 1 tablespoon fresh mint leaves
- 2 tablespoons fresh key lime juice
- ½ cup chilled spring water

Directions:

1. Combine all ingredients in a powerful blender, and mix until smooth.

2. Place in serving dishes, then serve immediately.

Nutrition:

Calories: 76 Fat: 0.1 g Carbs: 18.7 g Protein: 1.1 g

Strawberry Ice Cream

Preparation Time: 15 minutes
Cooking Time: 15 minutes
Servings: 6
Ingredients:

- 5 frozen burro bananas
- 1 cup frozen strawberries
- ½ of avocado; peeled, pitted, and chopped
- ¼ cup unsweetened hemp milk
- 1 tablespoon agave nectar

Directions:

1. Place all ingredients in a powerful blender, and mix until smooth.
2. Place the strawberry mixture in an airtight container and place in the fridge for a few hours, or until it becomes hard, before serving.

Nutrition:

Calories: 143 Fat: 0.8 g Carbs: 28.5 g Protein: 1.6 g

Lime Sorbet

Preparation Time: 10 minutes
Cooking Time: 10 minutes
Servings: 4
Ingredients:

- 2 tablespoons fresh key lime zest, grated
- ½ cup agave nectar
- 2 cups spring water
- 1½ cups fresh key lime juice

Directions:

1. Before creating this sorbet, freeze the ice cream machine tub for around 24 hours.
2. Over medium heat, combine all of the ingredients (apart from the lime juice) in a nonstick saucepan. Simmer, constantly stirring, for about 1 minute.

3. Turn off the heat and whisk in the lime juice to the mixture.

4. Place this in an airtight container and chill for about two hours.

5. Next, add the lime mixture to an ice cream machine and process it in accordance with the instructions provided by the manufacturer.

6. Place the ice cream back in the airtight container and freeze for around two hours.

Nutrition:

Calories: 130 Fat: 0 g Carbs: 33.4 g Protein: 0.1 g

Avocado Mousse

Preparation Time: 15 minutes

Cooking Time: 15 minutes

Servings: 4

Ingredients:

- 2 cups burro bananas, peeled and chopped
- 2 ripe avocados; peeled, pitted, and chopped
- 2 teaspoons fresh key lime zest, grated finely
- 1 cup fresh key lime juice
- 1/3–½ cup agave nectar

Directions:

1. Place all ingredients in a blender and mix on high until they are smooth and creamy.

2. Divide the mousse into four serving glasses and place in the fridge for approximately three hours to cool.

Nutrition:

Calories: 358 Fat: 4.2 g Carbs: 47.9 g Protein: 2.8 g

Grilled Peaches

Preparation Time: 10 minutes

Cooking Time: 6 minutes

Servings: 2

Ingredients:

- 2 large peaches, halved and pitted
- 1/8 teaspoon ground cinnamon
- 1 tablespoon walnuts, chopped

Directions:
1. Preheat the grill to medium-high heat.
2. Grease the grill grate.
3. Arrange the peach halves onto the prepared grill, cut side down and cook for about 3–5 minutes per side.
4. Remove the peach halves from grill and place onto serving plates.
5. Set aside to cool slightly.
6. Sprinkle with cinnamon and walnuts and serve.

Nutrition:
Calories: 83 Fat: 0.1 g Carbs: 14.5 g Protein: 2.4 g

Chickpea Mashed Potatoes

Preparation Time: 5 minutes
Cooking Time: 30 minutes
Servings: 4

Ingredients:
- 2 cups chickpeas, cooked
- ¼ cup green onions, diced
- 2 teaspoons sea salt
- 2 teaspoons onion powder
- 1 cup walnut milk; homemade, unsweetened

Directions:
1. Turn on the food processor, add the chickpeas and milk, and then season with salt and onion powder.
2. Put the lid on the blending jar and pulse for 1 to 2 minutes, or until the mixture is smooth; add water if necessary.
3. Place the blended chickpea mixture in a medium saucepan and cook it over medium heat.
4. Add green onions to the chickpea mixture and stir continuously for 30 minutes while the mixture cooks.

Nutrition:
Calories: 145.8 Carbs: 19.1g Fat: 7.3g Protein: 3.3g

Mushroom and Onion Gravy

Preparation Time: 5 minutes
Cooking Time: 18 minutes
Servings: 4
Ingredients:

- 1 cup sliced onions, chopped
- 1 cup mushrooms, sliced
- 2 teaspoons onion powder
- 2 teaspoons sea salt
- 1 teaspoon dried thyme
- 6 tablespoons chickpea flour
- ½ teaspoon cayenne pepper
- 1 teaspoon dried oregano
- 4 tablespoons grapeseed oil
- 4 cups spring water

Directions:
1. Heat oil in a medium saucepan over medium-high heat. Once heated, add the onions and mushrooms, and sauté for one minute.
2. Add salt, oregano, thyme, onion powder, and salt to the veggies. Cook for 5 minutes after thoroughly combining.
3. Add water, whisk in cayenne pepper, and then heat the mixture to a rolling boil.
4. Stir in the chickpea flour gradually and return the mixture to a boil.
5. Turn off the heat and serve the gravy with a favourite meal.
Nutrition:
Calories: 120 Carbs: 8.4g Fat: 7.6g Protein: 2.2g

Creamy Kale Salad With Avocado and Tomato

Preparation Time: 5 minutes
Cooking Time: 10 minutes
Servings: 2

Ingredients:

- 2 handful of kale
- 2 cherry tomatoes
- 1 ripe avocado
- Juice from 1 lime
- 1 garlic clove, crushed
- 1 tablespoon agave
- 1/2 tablespoon paprika
- 1/2 tablespoon black pepper

Directions:

1. Roughly cut the tomatoes and greens after washing them. Put them in a basin for mixing.
2. Add the avocado to the mixing bowl after peeling it.
3. Fill the bowl with the other ingredients and mix everything well before adding the lemon juice.
4. Present and savour.

Nutrition:

Calories: 179.2 Fat: 14.1g Carbs: 13.5g Protein: 3.7g

Vegetable Chili

Preparation Time: 5 minutes
Cooking Time: 30 minutes
Servings: 6

Ingredients:

- 2 cups black beans, cooked
- 1 medium red bell pepper; deseeded, chopped
- 1 poblano chili; deseeded, chopped
- 2 jalapeño chilies; deseeded, chopped

- 4 tablespoons cilantro, chopped
- 1 large white onion; peeled, chopped
- 1 ½ tablespoon minced garlic
- 1 ½ teaspoon sea salt
- 1 ½ teaspoon cumin powder
- 1 ½ teaspoon red chili powder
- 3 teaspoons lime juice
- 2 tablespoons grapeseed oil
- 2 ½ cups vegetable stock

Directions:

1. Place oil in a large saucepan over medium-high heat. When the oil is heated, add the onion and cook for 4–5 minutes, or until the onion is transparent.

2. Include the bell pepper, jalapeño pepper, poblano chile, and garlic. Cook the vegetables for 3–4 minutes, or until they are soft.

3. Salt the veggies, mix in the cumin and red chilli powder, add the chickpeas, and then add the vegetable stock.

4. Once the mixture comes to a boil, reduce the heat to medium-low, cover, and simmer the chilli for 15 to 20 minutes, or until it slightly thickens.

5. After that, turn off the heat, divide the chilli stew into six bowls, top with lime juice, add cilantro, and plate.

Nutrition:

Calories: 224.2 Carbs: 42.6g Fat: 1.2g Protein: 12.5g

Avocado Salad

Preparation Time: 10 minutes
Cooking Time: 5 minutes
Servings: 4

Ingredients:

- 1 avocado, finely chopped
- 3 tablespoons boiled corn

- 1 tomato, thinly chopped
- 1 tablespoon extra-virgin olive oil
- Salt to taste
- 1 tablespoon lemon juice
- 3 green onions, chopped

Directions:

1. Add the chopped avocado and lemon juice to a big bowl and stir.
2. Combine it with the other ingredients, except the tomato, in the same bowl.
3. Arrange sliced tomatoes on top of the dish.

Nutrition:

Calories: 164.2 Fat: 11.8g Carbs: 11.6g Protein: 5.4g

Wild Rice and Black Lentils Bowl

Preparation Time: 10 minutes

Cooking Time: 50 minutes

Servings: 4

Ingredients:

- Wild rice
- 2 cups wild rice, uncooked
- 4 cups spring water
- ½ teaspoon salt
- 2 bay leaves
- Black lentils
- 2 cups black lentils, cooked
- 1 ¾ cups coconut milk, unsweetened
- 2 cups vegetable stock
- 1 teaspoon dried thyme
- 1 teaspoon dried paprika
- ½ of medium purple onion; peeled, sliced
- 1 tablespoon minced garlic
- 2 teaspoons creole seasoning

- 1 tablespoon coconut oil
- Plantains
- 3 large plantains, chopped into ¼-inch-thick pieces
- 3 tablespoons coconut oil
- Brussels sprouts
- 10 large brussels sprouts, quartered
- 2 tablespoons spring water
- 1 teaspoon sea salt
- ½ teaspoon ground black pepper

Directions:

1. To start cooking the rice, use a medium saucepan and boil some water in it while adding salt and bay leaves.

2. After bringing the water to a boil, reduce the heat to medium, add the rice, and simmer for at least 30 to 45 minutes to make the rice soft.

3. After the rice is prepared, remove the bay leaves, drain any water that may still be in the pot, turn off the heat, and fluff with a fork. Put aside till required.

4. While the rice is cooking, prepare the lentils. In a large saucepan, heat the oil over medium-high heat. When the oil is heated, add the onion and simmer, stirring occasionally, for 5 minutes or until transparent.

5. Add the other ingredients for the lentils and toss to combine after cooking the onion and garlic together for 2 minutes, or until the garlic is fragrant and golden.

6. After bringing the lentils to a boil, reduce the heat to low, cover the pot with a lid, and simmer the lentils for 20 minutes, or until they are cooked.

7. When finished, turn off the heat and leave the pot aside.

8. Slice the plantains into 1/4-inch-thick slices and get the rice and lentils simmering.

9. Heat a large skillet over medium heat, add the coconut oil, and when it melts, add half of the plantain pieces. Cook, flipping

occasionally, for at least 7 to 10 minutes each side, or until golden brown.

10. After finished, remove the browned plantains from the pan and put them aside until required. Repeat with the remaining plantain pieces.

11. To prepare the sprouts, reheat the skillet over medium heat and, if necessary, add extra oil before adding the brussels sprouts.

12. Cook the sprouts for 3–4 minutes on each side, or until they are golden brown, after tossing them to coat them with oil.

13. Pour water over the sprouts, cover the pan with the lid, and steam for 3 to 5 minutes.

14. Add salt and black pepper to the sprouts, toss to combine, and then transfer to a platter.

15. Construct the dish by dividing the rice among the four bowls equally, followed by the lentils, plantain slices, and sprouts.

16. Present right away.

Nutrition:
Calories: 224.2 Carbs: 42.6g Fat: 1.2g Protein: 12.5g

Spaghetti Squash With Peanut Sauce

Preparation Time: 15 minutes
Cooking Time: 15 minutes
Servings: 4
Ingredients:

- 1 cup cooked shelled edamame; frozen, thawed
- 3-pound spaghetti squash
- ½ cup red bell pepper, sliced
- ¼ cup scallions, sliced
- 1 medium carrot, shredded
- 1 teaspoon minced garlic
- ½ teaspoon crushed red pepper
- 1 tablespoon rice vinegar

- ¼ cup coconut aminos
- 1 tablespoon maple syrup
- ½ cup peanut butter
- ¼ cup unsalted roasted peanuts, chopped
- ¼ cup and 2 tablespoons spring water, divided
- ¼ cup fresh cilantro, chopped
- 4 lime wedges

Directions:

1. To prepare the squash, slice each one in half lengthwise, then scoop out the seeds.

2. Place the squash halves cut-side up in a microwave-safe dish. Drizzle with 2 tablespoons of water. Microwave on high for 10-15 minutes, or until the squash is soft.

3. Let the squash to cool for 15 minutes before handling. To create noodles, scrape the meat of the animal lengthwise with a fork. After making noodles, let them cool for ten minutes.

4. While the squash is heating up in the microwave, make the sauce by whisking together the vinegar, coconut aminos, maple syrup, and water in a medium bowl with the butter, red pepper, and garlic.

5. Once the squash noodles have cooled, divide them equally among four bowls, top with bell pepper, carrots, edamame beans, and scallions, and then drizzle with the prepared sauce.

6. Top each dish with a lime slice and garnish with cilantro and peanuts.

Nutrition:

Calories: 419 Carbs: 32.8g Fat: 24g Protein: 17.6g

Kale Caesar Salad

Preparation Time: 5 minutes
Cooking Time: 12 minutes
Servings: 1

Ingredients:

- 1 bunch of curly kale, washed

- 1 cup sunflower seeds
- 1/3 cup almond nuts
- 1/8 tablespoon chipotle powder
- 2 garlic cloves
- 1-1/4 water
- 1-1/2 tablespoon agave syrup
- 1/2 tablespoon sea salt

Directions:
1. Wash the curly kale, pat it dry, and take the membrane out of the middle. Kale leaves should be torn into tiny pieces.
2. Place all remaining ingredients in a blender and process until creamy and smooth.
3. After adding half of the mixture, toss the kale to thoroughly coat it.
4. Pour the remaining liquid over the kales and stir to evenly coat the folds and curls.
5. After a 10-minute rest period, serve on plates. Add sunflower seeds, then have pleasure.

Nutrition:
Calories: 157 Fat: 6g Carbs: 18g Protein: 9g

Cauliflower Alfredo Pasta

Preparation Time: 10 minutes
Cooking Time: 30 minutes
Servings: 4

Ingredients:
- Alfredo sauce
- 4 cups cauliflower florets, fresh
- 1 tablespoon minced garlic
- ¼ cup nutritional yeast
- ½ teaspoon garlic powder
- ¾ teaspoon sea salt
- ½ teaspoon onion powder

- ½ teaspoon ground black pepper
- ½ tablespoon olive oil
- 1 tablespoon lemon juice, and more as needed for serving
- ½ cup almond milk, unsweetened
- Pasta
- 1 tablespoon minced parsley
- 1 lemon, juiced
- ½ teaspoon sea salt
- ¼ teaspoon ground black pepper
- 12 ounces spelt pasta; cooked, warmed

Directions:

1. Fill a large saucepan half full of water and heat it to a boil over medium-high heat.
2. Add the cauliflower florets, simmer for 10 to 15 minutes or until cooked, then remove and thoroughly drain.
3. Place a medium skillet over low heat, add the oil, and when it is heated, add the garlic. Cook the garlic for 4–5 minutes, or until it is aromatic and golden brown.
4. Place cauliflower florets and the additional ingredients for the sauce in a food processor. Pulse for 2 to 3 minutes, or until the mixture is smooth.
5. Pour the sauce into the pan, give it a good toss, and cook it for 5 minutes, or until it is hot.
6. Add the pasta to the saucepan, toss it well to coat it, check the seasoning, and simmer for 2 minutes or until the pasta is heated through.
7. Distribute the pasta and sauce among the four dishes, season with salt and pepper, squeeze the lemon juice over the top, and sprinkle the chopped parsley on top.

Nutrition:

Calories: 360 Carbs: 59g Fat: 9g Protein: 13g

Creamy Avocado Cilantro Lime Dressing

Preparation Time: 20 minutes
Cooking Time: 10 minutes
Servings: 6-8
Ingredients:

- ¼ cup olive oil
- ¼ teaspoon of sea salt
- ½ cup cilantro, chopped
- ¼ cup plain goat yogurt
- Juice of ½ lime
- 1 teaspoon lime zest
- 1 avocado
- 1 clove garlic, peeled
- ½ jalapeno, chopped
- ¼ teaspoon pepper
- ½ teaspoon cumin

Directions:

1. Combine all the ingredients in a food processor or mixer until they are evenly distributed.

Nutrition:

Calories: 123 Protein: 1g Fat: 12g Carbs: 3.6g

Side Dishes

Lettuce Salad

Preparation time: 5 minutes
Cooking time: 0 minutes
Servings: 4
Ingredients:

- 1 tablespoon ginger, grated
- 2 garlic cloves, minced
- 4 cups romaine lettuce, torn
- 1 beet, peeled and grated
- 2 green onions, chopped
- 1 tablespoon balsamic vinegar
- 1 tablespoon sesame seeds

Directions:

1. Toss the lettuce with the ginger, garlic, and other ingredients in a bowl before serving as a side dish.

Nutrition:

Calories: 42, Fat: 1.4, Carbs: 6.7, Protein: 1.4

Chives Radishes

Preparation time: 5 minutes
Cooking time: 0 minutes
Servings: 4
Ingredients:

- 1 pound red radishes, roughly cubed
- 1 tablespoon chives, chopped
- 1 tablespoon parsley, chopped
- 1 tablespoon oregano, chopped
- 2 tablespoons olive oil
- 1 tablespoon lime juice
- Black pepper to the taste

Directions:
1. Combine the radishes, chives, and other ingredients in a salad bowl; toss to combine; then serve.
Nutrition:
Calories: 85, Fat: 7.3, Carbs: 5.6, Protein: 1

Lime Fennel Mix
Preparation time: 5 minutes
Cooking time: 20 minutes
Servings: 4
Ingredients:

- 2 fennel bulbs, sliced
- 1 teaspoon sweet paprika
- 1 small red onion, sliced
- 2 tablespoons olive oil
- 2 tablespoons lime juice
- 2 tablespoons dill, chopped
- Black pepper to the taste

Directions:
1. Place the fennel, paprika, and other spices in a roasting pan, mix to incorporate, and bake for 20 minutes at 380 degrees F.
2. Distribute the mixture among dishes, then serve.
Nutrition:
Calories: 114, Fat: 7.4, Carbs: 13.2, Protein: 2.1

Oregano Peppers
Preparation time: 10 minutes
Cooking time: 30 minutes
Servings: 4
Ingredients:

- 1 pound mixed bell peppers, cut into wedges

- 1 red onion, thinly sliced
- 2 tablespoons olive oil
- Black pepper to the taste
- 1 tablespoon oregano, chopped
- 2 tablespoons mint leaves, chopped

Directions:

1. Place the bell peppers, onion, and other ingredients in a roasting pan, mix to incorporate, and bake for 30 minutes at 380 degrees F.

2. Distribute the mixture among dishes, then serve.

Nutrition:

Calories: 240, Fat: 8.2, Carbs: 11.3, Protein: 5.6

Red Cabbage Sauté

Preparation time: 5 minutes

Cooking time: 15 minutes

Servings: 4

Ingredients:

- 1 pound red cabbage, shredded
- 8 dates, pitted and sliced
- 2 tablespoons olive oil
- ¼ cup veggie stock
- 2 tablespoons chives, chopped
- 2 tablespoons lemon juice
- Black pepper to the taste

Directions:

1. In a medium-sized pan, heat the oil. Add the cabbage and dates; toss to combine; cook for 4 minutes.

2. Add the liquid and the other ingredients, mix, and simmer for an additional 11 minutes over medium-low heat before dividing amongst plates and serving.

Nutrition:

Calories: 280, Fat: 8.1, Carbs: 8.7, Protein: 6.3

Black Beans and Shallots Mix

Preparation time: 4 minutes

Cooking time: 0 minutes

Servings: 4

Ingredients:

- 3 cups black beans, cooked
- 1 cup cherry tomatoes, halved
- 2 shallots, chopped
- 3 tablespoons olive oil
- 1 tablespoon balsamic vinegar
- Black pepper to the taste
- 1 tablespoon chives, chopped

Directions:

1. Toss the beans, tomatoes, and other ingredients in a bowl and serve cold as a side dish.

Nutrition:

Calories: 310, Fat: 11.0, Carbs: 19.6, Protein: 6.8

Cilantro Olives Mix

Preparation time: 4 minutes

Cooking time: 0 minutes

Servings: 4

Ingredients:

- 2 spring onions, chopped
- 2 endives, shredded
- 1 cup black olives, pitted and sliced
- ½ cup kalamata olives, pitted and sliced
- ¼ cup apple cider vinegar
- 2 tablespoons olive oil
- 1 tablespoons cilantro, chopped

Directions:

1. Combine the endives with the remaining ingredients in a dish, stir, and serve.
Nutrition:
Calories: 230, Fat: 9.1, Carbs: 14.6, Protein: 7.2

Basil Tomatoes and Cucumbe r Mix
Preparation time: 5 minutes
Cooking time: 0 minutes
Servings: 4
Ingredients:
- ½ pound tomatoes, cubed
- 2 cucumber, sliced
- 1 tablespoon olive oil
- 2 spring onions, chopped
- Black pepper to the taste
- Juice of 1 lime
- ½ cup basil, chopped

Directions:
1. Place the tomatoes, cucumber, and other ingredients in a salad dish, stir, and serve chilled.
Nutrition:
Calories: 224, Fat: 11.2, Carbs: 8.9, Protein: 6.2

Peppers Salad
Preparation time: 5 minutes
Cooking time: 0 minutes
Servings: 4
Ingredients:
- 1 cup cherry tomatoes, halved
- 1 yellow bell pepper, chopped
- 1 red bell pepper, chopped

- 1 green bell pepper, chopped
- ½ pound carrots, shredded
- 3 tablespoons red wine vinegar
- 2 tablespoons olive oil
- 1 tablespoon cilantro, chopped
- Black pepper to the taste

Directions:

1. Toss the tomatoes, peppers, carrots, and the rest of the ingredients in a salad bowl before serving as a side salad.

Nutrition:

Calories: 123, Fat: 4, Carbs: 14.4, Protein: 1.1

Rice and Cranberries Mix

Preparation time: 10 minutes
Cooking time: 25 minutes
Servings: 4

Ingredients:

- 1 cup cauliflower florets
- 1 cup brown rice
- 2 cups chicken stock
- 1 tablespoon avocado oil
- 2 shallots, chopped
- ¼ cup cranberries
- ½ cup almonds, sliced

Directions:

1. Add the shallots to a pan with the oil already heated over medium heat. Stir and cook for 5 minutes.

2. Include the cauliflower, rice, and the other ingredients. Toss, bring to a simmer, and cook for 20 minutes on medium heat.

3. Distribute the mixture among dishes, then serve.

Nutrition:

Calories: 290, Fat: 15.1, Carbs: 7, Protein: 4.5

Oregano Beans Salad

Preparation time: 10 minutes
Cooking time: 0 minutes
Servings: 4

Ingredients:

- 2 cups black beans, cooked
- 2 cups white beans, cooked
- 2 tablespoons balsamic vinegar
- 2 tablespoons olive oil
- 1 teaspoon oregano, dried
- 1 teaspoon basil, dried
- 1 tablespoon chives, chopped

Directions:

1. Toss the beans with the vinegar and the other ingredients in a salad bowl and serve as a side salad.

Nutrition:

Calories: 322, Fat: 15.1, Carbs: 22.0, Protein: 7

Coconut Beets

Preparation time: 5 minutes
Cooking time: 20 minutes
Servings: 4

Ingredients:

- 1 pound beets, peeled and cubed
- 1 red onion, chopped
- 1 tablespoon olive oil
- ½ cup coconut cream
- 4 tablespoons non-Fat: yogurt
- 1 tablespoon chives, chopped

Directions:

1. Add the onion to a skillet that has been heated with oil over medium heat, stir, and cook for 4 minutes.

2. Stir in the beets, cream, and other ingredients. Cook for an additional 15 minutes over medium heat. Divide across plates and serve.

Nutrition:

Calories: 250, Fat: 13.4, Carbs: 13.3, Protein: 6.4

Roasted Sweet Potato

Preparation time: 10 minutes

Cooking time: 1 hour

Servings: 4

Ingredients:

- 3 tablespoons olive oil
- 2 sweet potatoes, peeled and cut into wedges
- 2 beets, peeled, and cut into wedges
- 1 tablespoon oregano, chopped
- 1 tablespoon lime juice
- Black pepper to the taste

Directions:

1. Place the sweet potatoes and beets on a baking sheet that has been prepared, add the other ingredients, stir, and bake for one hour at 375 degrees F. 2. Place on plates as a side dish after being divided.

Nutrition:

Calories: 240, Fat: 11.2, Carbs: 8.6, Protein: 12.1

Coconut Kale Sauté

Preparation time: 10 minutes

Cooking time: 15 minutes

Servings: 4

Ingredients:

- 2 tablespoons olive oil
- 3 tablespoons coconut aminos

- 1 pound kale, torn
- 1 red onion, chopped
- 2 garlic cloves, minced
- 1 tablespoon lime juice
- 1 tablespoon cilantro, chopped

Directions:

1. In a medium-sized pan, heat the olive oil. Add the onion and garlic, and cook for 5 minutes.

2. Stir in the greens and the other ingredients, simmer for 10 minutes over medium heat, then divide across plates and serve.

Nutrition:

Calories: 200, Fat: 7.1, Carbs: 6.4, Protein: 6

Allspice Carrots

Preparation time: 10 minutes

Cooking time: 20 minutes

Servings: 4

Ingredients:

- 1 tablespoon lemon juice
- 1 tablespoon olive oil
- ½ teaspoon allspice, ground
- ½ teaspoon cumin, ground
- ½ teaspoon nutmeg, ground
- 1 pound baby carrots, trimmed
- 1 tablespoon rosemary, chopped
- Black pepper to the taste

Directions:

1. Toss the carrots with the oil, lemon juice, and other ingredients in a roasting pan. Place in the oven for 20 minutes at 400 degrees F.

2. Distribute among plates and serve.

Nutrition:

Calories: 260, Fat: 11.2, Carbs: 8.3, Protein: 4.3

Lemony Dill Artichokes

Preparation time: 10 minutes
Cooking time: 20 minutes
Servings: 4

Ingredients:

- 2 tablespoons lemon juice
- 4 artichokes, trimmed and halved
- 1 tablespoon dill, chopped
- 2 tablespoons olive oil
- A pinch of black pepper

Directions:

1. Toss the artichokes with the lemon juice and the other ingredients in a roasting pan. Bake for 20 minutes at 400 degrees F.
2. Distribute among plates and serve.

Nutrition:

Calories: 140, Fat: 7.3, Carbs: 17.7, Protein: 5.5

Juices & Smoothies

Very Green Smoothie

Preparation time: 10 minutes
Cooking time: 1 minutes
Servings: 1
Ingredients:

- 1 cup pineapple, chopped
- 1 cup baby spinach, chopped
- 1 green apple, cored and chopped
- ½ cup Greek yoghurt

Directions:

1. In a blender or food processor, add the yoghurt, spinach, pineapple, and apple and pulse several times to incorporate and smooth out the mixture.
2. Pour into a cup and, if like, top with some pineapple pieces.
3. Place in a glass and sip.

Nutrition:
Calories 209; Fats 4g; Carbs 28g; Protein 8g

Reddy Anti-Inflammatory Smothie

Preparation time: 10 minutes
Cooking time: 1 minutes
Servings: 2
Ingredients:

- 1 cup strawberries, frozen and chopped
- ½ cup blueberries, frozen and chopped
- 1 medium beetroot, chopped
- 1 cup beet greens, chopped
- ½ cup raw orange juice

Directions:

1. Blend the beetroot greens and orange juice in a blender for one minute.

2. In a blender or food processor, add the diced strawberries, blueberries, and beets and process until smooth.

3.Add some berries as a garnish after pouring into a cup.

4. Pour into a glass and enjoy!

Nutrition:

Calories 190; Fats 4g; Carbs 25g; Protein 4g

Papaya smoothie

Preparation time: 10 minutes

Cooking time: 1 minutes

Servings: 2

Ingredients:

- 1 medium avocado, chopped
- 1 red apple, cored and chopped
- 1 cup ripe papaya chunks
- 2 tablespoons hazelnuts, roasted
- ½ cup almond milk

Directions:

1. In a blender or food processor, add the almond milk, hazelnuts, avocado, apple, and papaya. Pulse until well-combined and creamy in texture.

2. If extra almond milk is required, add it and blend until the mixture is smooth.

3. Pour into a cup and add some hazelnuts as a garnish.

4. Pour into a glass and enjoy!

Nutrition:

Calories 245; Fats 12g; Carbs 12g; Protein 4g

Broccoli Smoothie

Preparation time: 10 minutes

Cooking time: 1 minutes
Servings: 2
Ingredients:
- 1cup pineapple chunks
- 1 green apple, chopped
- 5 fingers carrots, chopped
- 1 broccoli head, chopped
- 1 teaspoon ground turmeric

Directions:
1. Blend for one minute after adding pineapple, Apple, carrots, and broccoli.
2. Place the ground turmeric in a blender or food processor, and pulse for two to three minutes, or until the mixture is smooth and creamy.
3. Place in a glass and sip.
Nutrition:
Calories 160; Fat 1g; Carbs 21g; Protein 3g

Raspberry Smoothie
Preparation time: 5 minutes
Cooking time: 1 minutes
Servings: 1
Ingredients:
- 1 cup raspberries, halved
- 1 small ripe banana, frozen and chopped
- 1 broccoli head, chopped
- 1 small beet, chopped
- ½ a lemon, juiced
- 2 scoops Greek yoghurt

Directions:
1. Blend some beetroot, broccoli, and banana in a blender for one minute.

2. In the blender or food processor, add the raspberries and yoghurt and pulse until well incorporated and smooth.
3. Add lemon juice and process until the mixture is smooth.
4. Pour into a cup and add some raspberries as a garnish.
5. Pour into a glass and enjoy!
Nutrition:
Calories: 260; Fat: 6g; Carbs: 35g; Protein: 10g

Watermelon Smoothie
Preparation time: 5 minutes
Cooking time: 1 minutes
Servings: 1
Ingredients:
- 1 cup watermelon, frozen and chopped
- 1 cup strawberries, frozen and chopped
- 2 teaspoons chia seeds, soaked
- 2 teaspoon honey
- 2 scoops of low-fat yoghurts

Directions:
1. First, soak the chia seeds in water for one whole night in a small basin.
2. In the blender or food processor, combine the soaked chia seeds with the yoghurt and puree for one minute.
3. In the blender or food processor, add the watermelon, strawberries, and honey and pulse until well-combined and creamy.
4. Pour into a glass cup and add some strawberries as a garnish.
5. Present and savour!
Nutrition:
Calories: 213; Fat: 4g; Carbs: 31g; Protein: 8g

Spinach Smoothie
Preparation time: 8 minutes
Cooking time: 1 minutes
Servings: 1

Ingredients:
- 1 cup spinach, chopped
- 5 cherry tomatoes, chopped
- 1 mango, chopped
- ½ ripe banana, chopped
- 1 cup coconut water

Directions:
1. In a blender or food processor, add some coconut water, spinach, tomatoes, mango, and banana. Pulse for approximately 3 to 5 minutes, or until everything is well-combined and creamy.
Pour the liquid into a glass to serve.

Nutrition:
Calories 196; Fat 5g; Carbs 30g; Protein 6g

Rolled-Oat Smoothie

Preparation time: 7 minutes
Cooking time: 1 minutes
Servings: 1

Ingredients:
- ½ cup rolled oats
- 1 cup blackberries
- 2 tablespoons Flax Seeds, roasted
- 1 ripe avocado, chopped
- 2 dates Medjool, pitted
- 1 cup almond milk

Directions:
1. Blend oats, dates, and flax seeds in a blender with a little almond milk for a minute.
2. Add the blackberries and avocado, which have been diced, to the blender or food processor, and pulse until well blended.
3. Pour into a cup and top with some flaxseeds and blackberries.
4. Pour into a glass and enjoy!

Nutrition:
Calories 28; Fat 15g; Carbs 38g; Protein 11g

Celery & Waternelon Juice
Preparation time: 9 minutes
Cooking time: 1 minutes
Servings: 1
Ingredients:
- 1 cup watermelon, chopped
- 1 cup strawberries, chopped
- 1 bunch of celery stalks, chopped
- ½ a lemon, freshly squeezed

Directions:
1. To disinfect them, wash all the fruits and vegetables under running water.
2. Cut into pieces and juice each piece separately in a small dish.
3. Incorporate the leftover solids into a smoothie or a soup.
4. Pour your juice into a jar, squeeze the lemon over over, and mix.
5. Handle chilled in a glass or whatever you choose.
Nutrition:
Calories 128; Fat 1g; Carbs 28g; Protein 3g

Apple Orange Juice
Preparation time: 10 minutes
Cooking time: 1 minutes
Servings: 1
Ingredients:
- 1 cup pineapple chunks, frozen
- 1 cup red grapes, frozen
- 1 red apple, cored and chopped
- 1 handful of mint leaves

- 1 fresh orange, juiced

Directions:

1. Thoroughly wash all the produce to remove any dirt.
2. Cut into pieces and juice each piece separately in a small dish.
3. To get the mint leaves through the juicer, juice the pineapple, apple, and grapes first, then the mint.
4. Use a citrus juicer to squeeze the orange juice into a glass.
5. Gather your juice using the juicer's nozzle into a container, then add the orange juice.
6. Include the leftover solids in a cake, smoothie, or soup.
7. Either serve your juice cold or right away.

Nutrition:

Calories 159; Fat 1g; Carbs 22g; Protein 2g

Cherry & Carrot Juice

Preparation time: 5 minutes
Cooking time: 1 minutes
Servings: 1

Ingredients:

- 1 cup ripe red cherries, pitted
- 1 cup carrots with greens
- 1-inch fresh turmeric, peeled and chopped
- 1 cup cucumber, chopped

Directions:

1. Run running water over all the fruits and vegetables.
2. After taking out the cherry's seeds, slice the remaining fruits and vegetables and juice them one at a time in a small dish.
3. Juice the pineapple and mint together, pushing the leaves through the juicer with the help of the pineapple.
4. Pour your juice into a glass, add the peeled turmeric, and serve right away.
5. Collect the residual sediments and include them into a smoothie or a soup dish.

Nutrition:
Calories: 180; Fat: 1g; Carbs: 19g; Protein: 1g

Beet & Grape Juice
Preparation time: 3 minutes
Cooking time: 1 minutes
Servings: 1
Ingredients:
- 1 bunch of celery, chopped
- 1 cup mixed grapes
- 1 medium beetroot
- 1 cup beet greens
- 1 cup pineapple chunks

Directions:
1. Wash the produce in a washbasin with running water.
2. Then, chop into smaller pieces in a basin, and juice each piece separately.
3. Juice the grapes and beetroot greens together to force the green leaves through the juicer.
4. Juice the pineapple, celery, and beets together. Strain the juice into a glass or jar using the juicer's nozzle, then chill it before serving.
5. Incorporate the leftover solids into a smoothie or a soup.
Nutrition:
Calories: 171; Fat: 1g; Protein: 2g Carbs: 25g

Merry Detox Juice
Preparation time: 6 minutes
Cooking time: 1 minutes
Servings: 1
Ingredients:
- 1 medium kiwifruit, chopped

- 1 medium pear, chopped
- 1 handful of coriander leaves, chopped
- 1 cup raspberries, halved
- 1-inch ginger

Directions:

1. Wash the produce in a washbasin with running water.

2. Cut into pieces and juice each piece separately in a small dish.

3. To force the coriander leaves through the juicer, combine the coriander and kiwifruit.

4. Squeeze the pear and raspberries, then add the ginger that has been peeled.

5. Incorporate the leftover solids into a smoothie or a soup.

6. Pour your juice into a glass or container and serve it cold or whichever you choose.

Nutrition:

Calories 171; Fat 2g; Carbs 26g; Protein 1g

Carrot & Apple Juice

Preparation time: 7 minutes

Cooking time: 1 minutes

Servings: 2

Ingredients:

- 1 grapefruit, segmented and deseeded
- 5 fingers baby carrots with greens
- 2 red apples, cored and chopped
- 1 cup pineapple chunks
- 1-inch ginger knob, peeled

Directions:

1. Start by giving all the produce a thorough wash under running water.

2. Peel the grapefruit, cut it into segments, and place it in a basin with no seeds.

3. In a small dish, chop up the remaining ingredients. Juice each piece separately.

4. Juice the apple and carrots together, pushing the vegetables through the juicer with the apple.

5. To make a flavorful juice, juice the pineapple, grapefruit, and ginger.

6. Blend the leftover particles with liquids or incorporate them into soups.

7. Put your juice in a container and serve it cold or whichever you choose.

Nutrition:

Calories 150; Fat 1g; Carbs 23g; Protein 2g

Very Berry Juice

Preparation Time: 5 minutes

Cooking Time: 1 minutes

Servings: 1

Ingredients:

- ½ strawberries halved
- ½ cup blackberries halved
- ½ cup raspberries halved
- ½ cup blueberries halved
- 1 small beet chopped
- 1 cup celery stalk, chopped
- ½ a lemon, freshly squeezed

Directions:

1. Start by giving all the produce a thorough wash under running water.

2. In a small bowl, cut the beetroot and celery and half the berries. Next, juice each piece separately.

3. Collect the residual solids and include them into a smoothie or a cake recipe.

4. Pour your juice into a jar, add some lemon juice, and top it off with a slice of lemon.

5. Enjoy by serving cold or as preferred!

Nutrition:

Calories: 137; Fat: 2g; Carbs: 19g; Protein: 3g

Blueberry Ginger Smoothie

Preparation time: 10 minutes

Cooking time: 0 minutes

Servings: 2

Ingredients:

- 2 cups blueberries
- 2 cups unsweetened almond milk
- 1 cup crushed ice
- ½ tsp ground ginger

Directions:

1. Use a blender to thoroughly combine all the ingredients. Dispense and savour!

Nutrition:

Calories: 125; Fat: 4g; Carbs: 23g; Protein: 2g

Conclusion

Fatty liver disease is a condition where there is an accumulation of fat in the liver, which can lead to inflammation, scarring, and even liver damage. It is a growing concern worldwide, and studies have shown that dietary changes can significantly improve the condition. A fatty liver diet cookbook can be a useful resource for people with fatty liver disease, providing them with guidance on what to eat and what to avoid to support liver health. In this conclusion, we will discuss the importance of a fatty liver diet, the benefits of following a fatty liver diet cookbook, and some key takeaways for individuals looking to improve their liver health.

The Importance of a Fatty Liver Diet

A fatty liver diet is essential for individuals with fatty liver disease because it can help to reduce inflammation, improve liver function, and prevent further liver damage. The liver is responsible for processing nutrients and removing toxins from the body. When the liver is compromised, it can affect overall health and well-being.

A healthy diet that supports liver health is one that is rich in whole foods, such as fruits, vegetables, whole grains, lean proteins, and healthy fats. A fatty liver diet cookbook can provide recipes and meal plans that are designed to help people with fatty liver disease make healthier food choices and support their liver health.

Benefits of Following a Fatty Liver Diet Cookbook

There are several benefits to following a fatty liver diet cookbook, including:

Improved Liver Health: A fatty liver diet cookbook can provide recipes that are low in fat and high in fiber, vitamins, and minerals, which can help to reduce inflammation, improve liver function, and prevent further liver damage.

Weight Management: Many people with fatty liver disease are overweight or obese, which can exacerbate the condition. A fatty liver diet cookbook can provide healthy meal plans and recipes that can help individuals achieve and maintain a healthy weight.

Reduced Risk of Complications: Fatty liver disease can lead to complications such as liver failure and liver cancer. A fatty liver diet cookbook can help individuals reduce their risk of these complications by providing them with healthy food options that support liver health.

Improved Quality of Life: Following a fatty liver diet cookbook can lead to an overall improvement in quality of life, as individuals may experience increased energy, improved mood, and better overall health.

Key Takeaways for Individuals with Fatty Liver Disease

Individuals with fatty liver disease can take several steps to support their liver health, including:

Eating a Healthy Diet: A healthy diet that supports liver health is one that is rich in whole foods, such as fruits, vegetables, whole grains, lean proteins, and healthy fats. A fatty liver diet cookbook can provide individuals with healthy meal plans and recipes that support liver health.

Exercise Regularly: Regular exercise can help individuals with fatty liver disease manage their weight, reduce inflammation, and improve liver function.

Limit Alcohol Consumption: Alcohol can exacerbate fatty liver disease and should be avoided or limited.

Avoid Processed Foods: Processed foods are typically high in fat, sugar, and salt and should be avoided as much as possible.

Work with a Healthcare Professional: Individuals with fatty liver disease should work with a healthcare professional to develop a comprehensive treatment plan that includes dietary changes, exercise, and other lifestyle modifications.

In conclusion, a fatty liver diet cookbook can be a valuable resource for individuals with fatty liver disease. It can provide them with guidance on what to eat and what to avoid to support liver health and improve overall health and well-being. By following a healthy diet, exercising regularly, limiting alcohol consumption, avoiding processed foods, and working with a healthcare professional, individuals with fatty liver disease can take steps to improve their liver health and reduce their risk of complications.

Made in United States
Orlando, FL
07 December 2024

55172068R00076